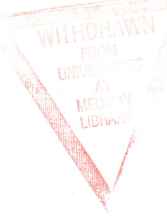
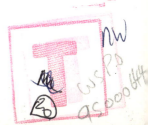

Biopsy Pathology of Muscle

BIOPSY PATHOLOGY SERIES

General Editors

Professor Leonard S. Gottlieb, MD, MPH
Mallory Institute of Pathology,
Boston, USA

Professor A. Munro Neville, PhD, DSc, MD, FRC Path.
Ludwig Institute for Cancer Research,
Zurich, Switzerland

Professor F. Walker, MD, PhD, FRC Path.
Department of Pathology,
University of Aberdeen, UK

Other titles in the series

Biopsy Pathology of Muscle

Second edition

MICHAEL SWASH
M.D. (London), F.R.C.P. (London), M.R.C. Path.
Consultant Neurologist, The Royal London Hospital
and St Mark's Hospital London,
and Senior Lecturer in Neuropathology,
The Medical College of the Royal London Hospital

and

MARTIN S. SCHWARTZ
M.D. (Maryland)
Consultant Clinical Neurophysiologist
St George's Hospital (Atkinson Morley's Hospital) London

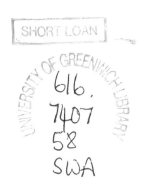

CHAPMAN & HALL MEDICAL
London · New York · Tokyo · Melbourne · Madras

UK	Chapman & Hall, 2–6 Boundary Row, London SE1 8HN
JAPAN	Chapman & Hall Japan, Thomson Publishing Japan, Hirakawacho Nemoto Building, 7F, 1-7-11 Hirakawa-cho, Chiyoda-ku, Tokyo 102
AUSTRALIA	Chapman & Hall Australia, Thomas Nelson Australia, 102 Dodds Street, South Melbourne, Victoria 3205
INDIA	Chapman & Hall India, R. Seshadri, 32 Second Main Road, CIT East, Madras 600 035

First edition 1984
Second edition 1991

© 1984, 1991 M. Swash and M.S. Schwartz

Typeset in 10/12pt Palatino by EJS Chemical Composition,
Midsomer Norton, Bath, Avon
Printed in Great Britain at the University Press, Cambridge

ISBN 0 412 34880 2

British Library Cataloguing in Publication Data

Swash, Michael 1939–
  Biopsy pathology of muscle.—2nd ed.
  1. Man. Muscles. Diagnosis. Biopsy
  I. Title II. Schwartz, Martin S. (Martin Samuel) III. Series
  616.740758
  ISBN 0–412–34880–2

Contents

vi   Contents

Acknowledgements

No book can be written without help from colleagues. We thank particularly Dr Jon van der Walt, Senior Lecturer in Morbid Anatomy at the Medical College of the Royal London Hospital, whose advice and help in updating Chapter 10, on tumours found in striated muscle, has been invaluable. Mr Ivor Northey in the department of medical photography of the Institute of Pathology at The London Hospital Medical College prepared the illustrations. The work which has led to the preparation of this book has been supported, at least in part, by The London Hospital Special Trustees, The Wellcome Trust, The Medical Research Council, The Motor Neuron Disease Association, and The London Hospital Medical College, and we gratefully acknowledge this support. Figure 2.2 was provided by Dr K.-G. Henriksson, Linkoping, Sweden, Fig. 2.7 by Professor Leo Duchen, Institute of Neurology, London, and Fig. 3.6 by Dr J.N. Cox, Cantonal Hospital, Geneva. We are particularly grateful to them for their help. A number of the illustrations are taken from our previous publications in various journals and these are reproduced here, with permission, as follows: Fig. 2.7, *Neurology*; Figs 4.12, 7.3, 7.5 and 8.6, *Journal of Neurology, Neurosurgery and Psychiatry*; Fig. 3.5a, b, *Journal of Anatomy*; Figs 4.12c, 6.17 and 8.4, *Brain*; Figs 4.3 and 8.14, *Muscle and Nerve*; Figs 4.6, 4.7, 5.7, 5.8, 5.14, 7.1, 7.8, 8.11 and 9.4 are reproduced from our book, *Neuromuscular Diseases: A Practical Approach to Diagnosis and Management*, Springer-Verlag, Berlin, Heidelberg, New York, 2nd edn (1988). Finally, we thank Mrs Adrienne Raine, who typed the manuscript with unfailing accuracy.

M. Swash
The Royal London Hospital, E1
M.S. Schwartz
Atkinson Morley's Hospital, SW20

Preface

Muscle biopsy is a long-established technique in clinical practice having been introduced by Duchenne in 1868 (*Arch. Gen. Med.*, **11**, 5–179). However, the needle method used by Duchenne was not generally adopted, although Shank and Hoagland described a similar technique in 1943 (*Science*, **98**, 592), and open muscle biopsy has for long been preferred in clinical practice, even with the advent of newer needle biopsy methods (Bergstrom, 1962, *Scand. J. Clin. Lab. Invest.*, **14**, Suppl. 68, 1–110). The development of enzyme histochemical techniques has contributed greatly to knowledge of muscle pathology. More recently electron microscopy and immunocytochemistry have also been applied to clinical diagnosis of neuromuscular disease.

This book is intended to serve as a practical guide in muscle pathology, particularly for histopathologists, and for those in training. As enzyme histochemistry has become more widely available, formalin-fixed methods have become less frequently used in muscle biopsy work.

In this new edition of *Muscle Biopsy Pathology* we have taken account of the advances in classification and histological technique, and in knowledge of neuromuscular diseases, that have emerged since the first edition was published in 1984. We hope that this book will continue to be used as a practical guide in the diagnosis and understanding of these disorders.

1. Introduction

1.1 General features of muscle

The differentiation of muscle into red and white types is a feature of all vertebrates and, indeed, of chordates. Red muscles are slow-contracting and specialized for postural activity, containing plentiful lipid droplets and mitochondria. White muscles, on the other hand, are faster contracting, suitable for short bursts of intense activity, but fatigue rapidly. They contain few lipid droplets and mitochondria, but plentiful glycogen granules. In man these fibre types are not found exclusively in individual muscles but occur in a random mosaic distribution in all muscles. The proportions of red and white muscle fibres in human muscles differ not only from muscle to muscle, but in relation to each individual's genetic characteristics. Although these two types of muscle fibre can be recognized in haematoxylin and eosin preparations of transverse sections of paraffin-embedded muscle, they can more easily be identified by the reciprocal relationship of their content of oxidative and non-oxidative enzymes (see Table 2.3). The red fibres react strongly for oxidative enzymes, e.g. succinic dehydrogenase, and are designated *Type 1 fibres*, and the white fibres react strongly for non-oxidative enzymes, e.g. myophosphorylase, and are designated *Type 2 fibres* (Dubowitz and Pearse, 1960).

The muscle fibres found in muscle spindles (intrafusal muscle fibres) and the muscle fibres in external ocular muscles, in other branchial muscles such as the masseter and facial muscles, and in the diaphragm and striated sphincter muscles, show striking differences in fibre-type distribution, fibre size, and even in their enzyme content when compared with the extrafusal, skeletal muscles that make up the bulk of the muscular system in limbs and trunk. Smooth muscle and cardiac muscle fibres are markedly different structures both in their morphological and functional characteristics.

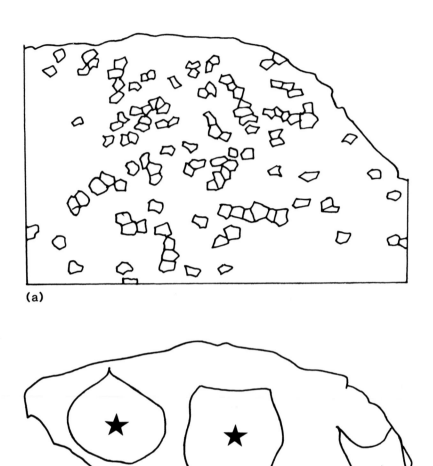

(a)

(b)

Fig. 1.1 (a) The muscle fibres belonging to a single motor unit are distributed quasi-randomly through part of the muscle. This drawing of the cross-sectional plane of a cat soleus muscle is taken from the work of Edstrom and Kugelberg (1968). The motor unit was identified by glycogen depletion after supramaximal stimulation of a single efferent nerve fibre in the appropriate ventral root. (b) Drawing of the territories of three separate motor units in a transverse section of the cat soleus (after Edstrom and Kugelberg, 1968).

1.2   The motor unit

Each mature extrafusal skeletal muscle fibre is innervated by a single nerve fibre, which terminates in a single motor end-plate. The functional unit in muscle, termed the motor unit by Sherrington, consists of a single anterior horn cell situated in the grey matter of the spinal cord, the motor axon derived from this cell, and its terminal branches, innervating a number of muscle fibres. The muscle fibres making up any individual motor unit are distributed through up to 30% of the cross-sectional area of a muscle (Fig. 1.1), in several fascicles. The fibres of one motor unit are therefore intermingled with other muscle fibres belonging to other motor units (Edstrom and Kugelberg, 1968; Brandstater and Lambert, 1973). The individual motor units cannot be recognized in specimens of muscle without special physiological/pathological correlation techniques.

Muscle fascicles (Fig. 1.2) are separated from each other by connective tissue which itself contains neurovascular bundles. Muscle spindles are situated in close association with these neurovascular bundles. The fascicular pattern of individual muscles varies. The length of muscle fibres in different muscles varies greatly, from a few millimetres to as much as 40 cm. Within a fascicle the muscle fibres are arranged in parallel, but individual fascicles are not usually arranged in the plane of the long axis of a muscle, but in a bipennate distribution inserting into a centrally situated tendinous plane. This arrangement may or may not be symmetrical, and there is great variability between different muscles. Golgi tendon organs are found in the major tendinous insertions and origins of muscles. The nerve supplying a muscle usually enters it, with its accompanying blood vessels, near the mid-point of the muscle.

The pathological features of diseases of muscle are determined by the disease process itself, by the intrinsic properties of muscle and by the close structural/functional relationship of muscle and its nerve supply. Thus diseases of muscle are broadly classified into *myopathies*, in which the disorder primarily affects the muscle fibres, and *neurogenic disorders*, in which muscular abnormalities result from disturbance of the innervation. By historical convention certain inherited myopathies are classified as *muscular dystrophies*, a term which implies a progressive course with marked change in the normal structure of the muscles.

1.3   Classification of neuromuscular disorders

There are a large number of different disorders in which muscle may be affected but, in the majority of these, muscle biopsy is not a useful investigation since it does not provide specific diagnostic information, and a diagnosis can be obtained more easily by other methods. For

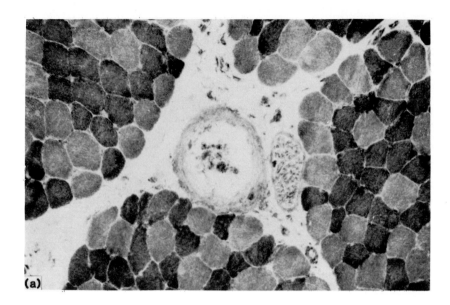

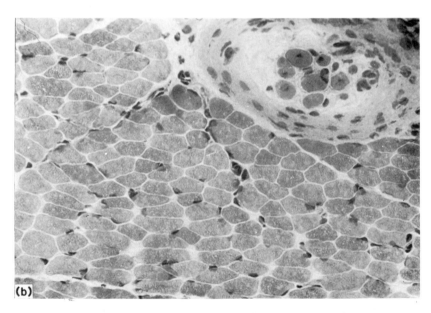

Fig. 1.2 (a) × 140; NADH. Normal muscle. A muscle spindle is seen in the interfascicular plane at the junction of several fascicles in the centre of the illustration, close to a small intramuscular nerve and a blood vessel – the neurovascular bundle. Two fibre types can be identified in the extrafusal muscle fibres; the intrafusal muscle fibres are very small and react intensely in this technique. (b) × 350; HE. Normal muscle spindle in a muscle biopsy from an infant. The intrafusal and extrafusal muscle fibres are approximately equal in size.

example, peripheral neuropathies, in which marked abnormalities occur in affected muscle, are usually diagnosed by clinical and electro-physiological techniques, and occasionally by nerve biopsy. In addition, many of the disorders noted in comprehensive classifications of neuro-muscular disorders are rare. The classification given here (Table 1.1) includes those disorders likely to be encountered in the pathological laboratory. A more complete classification is available (Walton and Gardner-Medwin, 1988). The most common condition in which muscle biopsy is likely to be performed is polymyositis, but this is not the commonest neuromuscular disorder; for example diabetic poly-neuropathy is far more frequent.

Table 1.1 A classification of neuromuscular disorders (modified from Swash and Schwartz, 1988)

MYOPATHIC DISORDERS

1. *Inflammatory myopathies*
   (a) *Idiopathic*
   Polymyositis
   Dermatomyositis
   Childhood dermatomyositis
   Polymyositis and dermatomyositis associated with carcinoma
   Polymyositis and dermatomyositis associated with collagen–vascular disease
   Granulomatous polymyositis (sarcoidosis)
   Eosinophilic polymyositis
   Inclusion-body myositis

   (b) *Infections*
   Viral
   Bacterial
   Infestations

2. *Drug-induced myopathies*

3. *Endocrine myopathies*
   Thyroid myopathies
   Osteomalacia and parathyroid disease
   Acromegalic myopathy
   Steroid myopathy

4. *Genetically determined myopathies*
   (a) *Muscular dystrophies*
   Duchenne muscular dystrophy
   Becker muscular dystrophy
   Limb-girdle muscular dystrophy
   Facioscapulohumeral muscular dystrophy
   Scapuloperoneal syndrome
   Oculopharyngeal muscular dystrophy
   Ocular myopathy

(b) *Myotonic syndromes*
   Myotonic dystrophy
   Myotonia congenita
   Other myotonic syndromes

(c) *Metabolic myopathies*
   Glycogenoses, e.g. McArdle's disease
   Lipid storage diseases, e.g. carnitine deficiency
   Mitochondrial myopathies
   Periodic paralyses
   Malignant hyperpyrexia
   Myoglobinurias

(d) *Myopathies of childhood*
   Central core and multicore disease
   Myotubular myopathy
   Nemaline myopathy
   Congenital fibre-type disproportion
   Congenital muscular dystrophy
   Other rare syndromes

NEUROGENIC DISORDERS

1. *Disorders of anterior horn cells*
   Spinal muscular atrophy (SMA)
     Type 1 Werdnig–Hoffmann disease
     Type 2 Intermediate SMA
     Type 3 Juvenile-onset Kugelberg–Welander disease
     Type 4 Adult-onset
   Motor neuron disease
   Poliomyelitis
   Other anterior horn cell disorders

2. *Disorders of motor nerve roots*
   Cervical and lumbar spondylosis with root compression
   Malignant infiltration of nerve roots
   Brachial neuritis (neuralgic amyotrophy)

3. *Peripheral neuropathies*
   (a) *Acquired polyneuropathies*
     (i) *metabolic*
        Diabetes mellitus
        Alcoholic neuropathy
        Renal and hepatic disease
        Vitamin deficiencies, e.g. B_{12} deficiency
     (ii) *Inflammatory polyradiculoneuropathy* (Guillain–Barré syndrome)
     (iii) *Drug-induced and toxic neuropathies*
        e.g. tri-ortho-cresyl phosphate poisoning, isoniazid neuropathy
     (iv) *Associated with malignant disease and paraproteinaemias*
     (v) *Infections*, e.g. leprosy, diphtheria
     (vi) *Associated with collagen vascular disease*
        e.g. polyartertis nodosa and other vasculitides, rheumatoid arthritis

(b) *Acquired mononeuropathies*
   Entrapment and compressive, e.g. carpal tunnel syndrome
   Trauma
   Mononeuritis multiplex

(c) *Genetically determined polyneuropathies*
   Charcot–Marie–Tooth syndrome
   Hereditary sensory neuropathies
   Amyloid neuropathy
   Other neuropathies with known metabolic defects,
       e.g. porphyria, metachromatic leucodystrophy, Refsum's disease

4. *Disorders of neuromuscular transmission* (end-plate disorders)
   Myasthenia gravis
   Myasthenic syndromes

1.4   Indications for muscle biopsy

Most muscle biopsies are arranged by rheumatologists, physicians, neurologists, or paediatricians. Rheumatologists and physicians are concerned particularly with patients with inflammatory muscle disease, usually associated with autoimmune disorders; neurologists use muscle biopsies for a wide variety of neuromuscular disorders, and paediatricians are involved with a different group of disorders, especially 'floppy baby' syndromes, muscular dystrophy and childhood-type dermatomyositis. These different specialists use muscle biopsy for somewhat different purposes.

   The main indications for muscle biopsy are shown in Table 1.2. Of these the most common are in the diagnosis of inflammatory muscle disease and in the diagnosis of proximal weakness of unknown cause. In relation to the frequency of muscle biopsy for these indications, biopsies in infants and children are rare except in specialized centres, since the childhood myopathies and dystrophies are relatively uncommon disorders. In general, muscle biopsies in patients with suspected autoimmune vasculitis are unlikely to provide useful information unless the muscle biopsied is clinically involved, either by tenderness or by weakness. Muscle biopsies in patients with metabolic myopathies, e.g. glycogenoses or mitochondrial cytopathies, are useful not only in providing a diagnosis of the clinical disorder, based on the histological appearances of the abnormal muscle, but in providing fresh tissue for biochemical and enzymatic analysis. Occasionally muscle biopsy studies are used in genetic analysis of risk in relatives of patients with a familial neuromuscular disorder.

Table 1.2   Indications for muscle biopsy

1. Inflammatory muscle disease before beginning treatment.
2. Proximal weakness of uncertain cause whether myopathic or neurogenic in adults and children, including 'floppy baby' syndromes.
3. Hereditary myopathies and muscular dystrophies.
4. To exclude treatable disorder, e.g. polymyositis, in patients in whom motor neuron disease is suspected.
5. Suspected metabolic myopathies, particularly in patients with muscle cramps, stiffness or tenderness.
6. Autoimmune vasculitis, especially polyarteritis nodosa, even in the absence of muscular symptoms.
7. Other systemic disorders, e.g. sarcoidosis, infestations.
8. To assess the effects of steroid treatment in the management of polymyositis, particularly in relation to the development of steroid myopathy.
9. Occasionally in carrier detection in female siblings or other close female relatives of boys with Duchenne dystrophy.
10. Diagnosis of malignant hyperpyrexia syndrome by *in vitro* test.
11. Research; e.g. exercise physiology, pathological and immunological studies, etc.

1.5   Selection of muscle for biopsy

Most biopsies are taken from the deltoid, biceps brachii or quadriceps femoris muscles, but triceps and gastrocnemius muscles are sometimes chosen if these muscles are considered more likely to show abnormality. Generally deltoid, biceps brachii and quadriceps femoris muscles are preferred for biopsy because no disability is likely to result from the biopsy. In addition, skin sutures are not under tension, the biopsy can be easily orientated for precise transverse and longitudinal sections, and the normal features of these muscles are well understood. The biceps brachii is particularly suitable because it contains approximately equal numbers of the different histochemical types of muscle fibre. In both deltoid and quadriceps femoris muscles there are variations in fibre-type proportions in different parts of the muscle. Occasionally, a muscle may be selected for biopsy because it is known from clinical, ultrasound or CT studies that it is particularly involved by the disease process (Schwartz *et al.*, 1988).

Muscles previously used for EMG should not be used for muscle biopsy because artefact caused by the needle electrode may lead to difficulty in interpretation. Indeed, marked abnormalities (needle myopathy) have been described (Engel, 1967). It is important to biopsy a muscle which is clinically affected, but muscles showing marked wasting should be avoided, since only end-stage fibrosis and fat replacement may be found. Generally, in neurogenic disorders moderately weak muscles should be biopsied whenever possible, but in myopathic conditions less severely involved muscles often show characteristic abnormalities and the choice of muscle is thus less important. In inflammatory muscle disease tender muscles are particularly likely to yield diagnostic information.

The development of needle muscle biopsy and of conchotome muscle biopsy (see Chapter 2) has encouraged clinicians to consider muscle biopsy in patients in whom open muscle biopsy would not be undertaken, and has allowed repeat biopsies to be undertaken when necessary. These techniques can sometimes be used in conjunction with open biopsy of an arm muscle to compare the distribution of abnormality in the upper and lower limbs.

1.6   Clinical features of neuromuscular disease

In the majority of patients in whom muscle biopsy is performed, the major problem is *weakness*. In most primary disorders of muscle, i.e. the myopathies, weakness is predominantly *proximal*, affecting the pelvic girdle muscles more severely than the shoulder girdle muscles. There is a characteristic waddling gait. Proximal weakness is also a feature of spinal muscular atrophy, a disorder in which muscular weakness and atrophy develops as a result of progressive loss of anterior horn cells. In some peripheral neuropathies in which there is involvement of spinal roots as well as of the peripheral nerves, e.g. Guillain–Barré polyradiculo-neuropathy, proximal weakness may also occur but, in general, peripheral neuropathies are characterized by *distal* weakness, which is usually symmetrical, and distal sensory loss or paraesthesiae. This distal weakness leads to footdrop and a high-stepping gait. In peripheral neuropathies the tendon reflexes are often absent, particularly the ankle jerks and, if present, muscular atrophy is also characteristically distal. In myopathies the tendon reflexes are usually present, although in Duchenne dystrophy, and in myotonic dystrophy, they are often reduced. In peripheral neuropathy the superficial nerves are sometimes enlarged, or tender.

In most inherited myopathies and dystrophies, *proximal weakness* is symmetrical, but particular muscle groups are often selectively involved. For example, in Duchenne dystrophy, weakness of the hip flexors and extensors, quadriceps and tibialis anterior is often prominent. In limb-girdle muscular dystrophy the biceps and periscapular muscles are particularly weak and in facioscapulohumeral muscular dystrophy, facial, triceps, biceps and periscapular muscles are mainly affected. Other rare variants, such as scapulo-peroneal atrophy and quadriceps myopathy, are recognized. In myotonic dystrophy facial and distal limb weakness, also involving small hand muscles, is characteristic, and there is marked weakness and atrophy of neck flexor muscles.

Pseudohypertrophy, a clinical phenomenon in which weak muscles appear enlarged and unusually firm to palpation, is a particular feature of Duchenne dystrophy, in which it especially involves periscapular, deltoid and gastrocnemius muscles, but it also occurs in some patients with limb-girdle dystrophy and, rarely, in hypothyroid myopathy, in certain other metabolic myopathies and in neurogenic disorders, e.g. root disorders. Involvement of the bulbar musculature is characteristic of myasthenia gravis and motor neuron disease. It also occurs in myotonic dystrophy and in the rare disorder, oculopharyngeal dystrophy, but it is uncommon in other myopathies.

Muscular wasting is a feature of most progressive myopathies, and usually occurs in the distribution of the weakness. Wasting is also a feature of neurogenic disorders. In the latter wasting may be accompanied by spontaneous fasciculation. This is an important and diagnostic feature of motor neuron disease, but it also occurs in some patients with spinal root lesions and, rarely, in thyrotoxicosis. In spinal muscular atrophies spontaneous fasciculation is uncommon, but fasciculation may occur after exercise and coarse tremulous contraction of individual muscle bundles can be recognized. In Werdnig–Hoffmann disease (infantile spinal muscular atrophy), however, fasciculation occurs at rest, especially in the tongue, even during sleep.

Myotonia consists of persistent contraction of a muscle or of part of a muscle after cessation of voluntary contraction. It can be recognized by its characteristic electromyographic features. It is usually a familial disturbance and may occur as an isolated clinical finding (e.g. myotonia congenita) or in association with other features of neuromuscular disease as in myotonic dystrophy or periodic paralysis.

Fatiguability is a common symptom noted not only by patients with neuromuscular diseases, but by patients with depression and as a reaction to undue psychological stress. It is thus difficult to define unless it is accompanied by definite evidence of a decrease in effort tolerance, or by the development of objective muscular weakness during exertion or movement. Fatiguability is particularly associated with myasthenia gravis. In this disorder weakness can usually be demonstrated by clinical tests of individual muscles during tonic or repeated movement. Commonly used tests include fist-clenching, abduction of the shoulder, and prolonged upward gaze leading to ptosis, but bulbar weakness is often evident during prolonged conversation or chewing. Fatiguability is also a feature of motor neuron disease, and of certain metabolic myopathies, particularly the mitochondrial myopathies. In polymyositis fatiguability is also a common complaint, especially in the early stages. Fatiguability is a feature of the post-viral syndrome.

Muscular pain and stiffness occurs in inflammatory myopathies, in which it is particularly prominent in the mornings, or after rest, and may be particularly relieved by exercise. Similar symptoms occur in patients with inflammatory joint disease and it may be difficult for the clinician to be certain whether or not there is muscular involvement in such cases. Muscular pain is a particularly prominent feature of polymyalgia rheumatica, although weakness is usually only slight in this condition. Muscular pain also occurs in certain metabolic myopathies, especially myxoedema and McArdle's syndrome (myophosphorylase deficiency). In these patients muscular pain, stiffness or cramp usually develops during exercise, although it may be relieved with continued exercise. In neurogenic disorders, including peripheral neuropathies, muscular pain is unusual. However, cramps at rest and with exercise are common in motor neuron disease, and severe muscular pain and tenderness may occur in Guillain–Barré syndrome and in alcoholic neuropathy.

Many neuromuscular diseases are accompanied by features of *involvement of other organs*. For example, in inflammatory myopathies there may be skin or joint involvement, in myotonic dystrophy cataract, diabetes mellitus and other features may coexist, in Duchenne dystrophy cardiac involvement is common, and in certain hereditary neuropathies pes cavus and other skeletal deformities are often found. These additional features may lead to recognition of the hereditary nature of the disorder. Careful enquiry about a possible family history is always important in the diagnosis of neuromuscular disorders.

The *age of onset* of symptoms is also important in diagnosis. In general, most hereditary conditions have specific patterns of presentation and progression and these can be readily recognized by experienced clinicians.

1.7   Clinical investigation of neuromuscular disorders

A wide variety of different tests can be used to assess patients with neuromuscular disorders but most of these are applicable only in rare instances. For example, the ischaemic lactate test is used in the diagnosis of McArdle's myophosphorylase deficiency; a low blood potassium level, often induced by exercise or by a glucose load, is important in the diagnosis of hypokalaemic periodic paralysis; various quantitative biochemical assays are used in the diagnosis of metabolic myopathies; thyroid function tests are useful in thyrotoxic and hypothyroid myopathies; tests for myoglobinuria may be helpful on some occasions; and measurement of serum immunoglobulins can be used in the diagnosis of some inflammatory myopathies, paraprotein-associated neuropathies, and polyarteritis. However, the most useful laboratory test is the measurement of *'muscle enzyme'* levels in the blood.

Although a number of different enzymes may be released from muscle in neuromuscular diseases, only aldolase, pyruvate kinase, carbonic anhydrase (CA III), and creatine kinase (CK) levels are useful in diagnosis. CK levels are usually preferred, since they provide a more sensitive indication of active muscular disease. The CK level is raised when muscle breakdown occurs, or when the muscle fibre membranes are abnormal, as in Duchenne dystrophy, allowing the muscle CK_{MM} isoenzyme to leak from the muscle cells into the circulation. In most laboratories CK isoenzyme assays are not available and the total venous blood CK level is measured. It is sometimes important to recognize that CK levels are affected by exercise and by the phase of the menstrual cycle.

Since the CK level varies with the extent of muscle fibre damage, and with the muscle bulk, the level tends to be highest in the early and most active stages of a disease, and to be lowest at the end-stage, when there is marked muscle atrophy. The CK level is also relatively low during healing stages of inflammatory myopathies, and it may fall during steroid therapy, even if the disease remains active. In metabolic myopathies the CK level is usually normal since muscle destruction is not a feature of these disorders; if muscle fibre necrosis occurs, as in McArdle's disease, the CK level may be transiently raised. In neurogenic disorders the CK level is usually normal, but it may be slightly raised in chronic neurogenic disorders.

In the past, 24-hour urinary creatine/creatinine ratios were used for the diagnosis of progressive muscular disorders as an index of muscle bulk and muscle cell necrosis, but they are now little used. Recently, the 24-hour urinary 3-methylhistidine excretion has been used as a measure of muscle catabolism.

An increasing number of genetic neuromuscular disorders have been localized to specific genetic loci, and these can be recognized by specific probes.

Electrocardiography is an important investigation since it provides evidence of an associated cardiomyopathy, e.g. in Duchenne dystrophy, myotonic dystrophy and Friedreich's ataxia.

Muscles may be *imaged* by ultrasonography, CT scanning or magnetic resonance imaging (MRI). These techniques provide measurements of size and of the extent of involvement of individual muscles.

Electromyography (EMG) is much used in the diagnosis of myopathic and neurogenic disorders. The technique consists both of needle electrode sampling of electrical activity in muscles at rest and during slight, graded muscular contraction, and of measurement of motor and sensory nerve conduction velocities. In the investigation of proximal weakness, the commonest presenting feature of patients submitted to muscle biopsy, needle EMG is particularly useful. Spontaneous electrical activity in resting muscle is uncommon except in neurogenic disorders, in which *fibrillations* representing spontaneous contractions of denervated muscle fibres, and *fasciculations*, representing spontaneous firing of parts or all of a motor unit, may occur. Fibrillations also occur rarely in myopathic disorders, in which segmental muscle necrosis may cause denervation of part of a muscle fibre by separating it from its nerve supply. Myotonic discharges can also be recognized during electrode insertion or movement.

During voluntary activation of a muscle the electrophysiological features of individual motor unit action potentials can be recognized, and the pattern and extent of their recruitment during increased activation can be studied. In neurogenic disorders individual potentials are larger and more complex than normal, owing to enlargement of the motor unit by reinnervation from axonal sprouts derived from surviving motor units. In myopathic disorders, however, individual potentials are smaller than normal, and usually shorter in duration, although they may also show increased complexity. This is due to loss of individual muscle fibres within the motor unit and to changes in muscle fibre size. The latter causes increased variability in the speed of propagation of the action potential in individual fibres.

In myasthenia gravis the abnormality of neuromuscular transmission at the motor end-plates results in fatiguability, which can be studied electrophysiologically. The size of the muscle action potential during repetitive stimulation of its nerve is progressively reduced in most myasthenic patients. In single-fibre EMG the variability in timing of the onset of depolarization in two or more muscle fibres belonging to a single motor unit is measured (the neuromuscular jitter), and is used as an index of the safety factor for neuromuscular transmission at the motor end-plates innervating these fibres. This diagnosis can also be made by assay of circulating acetylcholine receptor antibodies.

Nerve conduction studies are especially useful in the diagnosis of peripheral neuropathies, and may help differentiate neuropathies that are predominantly *axonal* in type from those that are predominantly *demyelinating*. They are particularly used in the diagnosis and management of entrapment neuropathies. Nerve conduction studies are usually normal in anterior horn cell disorders.

1.8   Animal models of human neuromuscular disease

Myopathic and neurogenic diseases, often resembling diseases of humans, occur in animals. Most of these have been recognized in other mammals, but avian myopathies also occur. Spinal muscular atrophy occurs in the Brittany spaniel, dystrophin deficiency muscular dystrophy occurs in the Mdx mouse (a model of Duchenne dystrophy), myotonia congenita occurs in the Tennessee myotonic goat, a glycogen storage disease resembling Pompe's Type II glycogenosis occurs in the Corriedale sheep and in the Shorthorn ox, and mitochondrial myopathies have been recognized in dogs (Bradley et al., 1988). These disorders are important both in veterinary practice and in the investigation of the disease processes underlying human neuromuscular disorders.

References

Bradley, R., McKerrell, R.E. and Barnard, E.A. (1988) Neuromuscular disease in animals. In Disorders of Voluntary Muscle, 5th edn (ed. J.N. Walton), Churchill Livingstone, Edinburgh, pp. 910–980.

Brandstater, M.E. and Lambert, E.G. (1973) Motor unit anatomy. In New Developments in Electromyography and Clinical Neurophysiology, Vol. 1 (ed. J.E. Desmedt), Karger, Basel, pp. 14–22.

Dubowitz, V. and Pearse, A.G.E. (1960) Reciprocal relationship of phosphorylase and oxidative enzymes in skeletal muscle. Nature, 185, 701.

Edstrom, L. and Kugelberg, E. (1968) Histochemical composition, distribution of fibres and fatiguability of single motor units. J. Neurol. Neurosurg. Psychiatry, 31, 424–433.

Engel, W.K. (1967) Focal myopathic changes produced by electromyographic and hypodermic needles. Arch. Neurol., 16, 509–513.

Schwartz, M.S., Swash, M., Ingram, D.A. et al. (1988) Patterns of selective involvement of thigh muscles in neuromuscular disease. Muscle Nerve, 11, 1240–1246.

Swash, M. and Schwartz, M.S. (1988) Neuromuscular Diseases: A Practical Approach to Diagnosis, 2nd edn, Springer-Verlag, London, pp. 456.

Walton, J.N. and Gardner-Medwin, D. (1988) Classification of neuromuscular disease. In Disorders of Voluntary Muscle, 5th edn (ed. J.N. Walton), Churchill Livingstone, Edinburgh.

2 The muscle biopsy: techniques and laboratory methods

There are several techniques available for muscle biopsy. Each has particular advantages and disadvantages and it is important for the pathologist to be aware of these (Table 2.1).

Open biopsy is carried out by a surgeon in the operating theatre, usually under local anaesthesia, but *needle biopsy* (Fig. 2.1, 2.2) can be performed at any convenient location (Edwards, 1971). Conchotome biopsy provides a slightly larger specimen than that available from needle biopsy (Fig. 2.2) (Henriksson, 1979). In order to obtain a specimen free of artefact and thus suitable both for light and electron microscopy it is important to maintain a scrupulous technique in handling the biopsy. In the case of open muscle biopsy the surgeon and his assistants must be aware that clamping, stretching, squeezing or drying the muscle tissue will all lead to unacceptable artefacts which may well interfere with proper interpretation of the biopsy. Muscle obtained by open biopsy should therefore be delivered to the waiting technician in the operating theatre so that the specimen can be dealt with immediately. Needle biopsy carries with it the advantage that the biopsy specimen is protected within the needle and is not therefore likely to be handled before it is given to the technician. Another source of artefact is the injection of local anaesthetic deeply into the muscle at the biopsy site. This results in disruption of the muscle tissue. Local anaesthetic should therefore only be injected into the skin and subcutaneous tissue. Since the perimysium contains pain fibres the incision or needle thrust into the muscle will, inevitably, be slightly painful, but this is a penalty that should be accepted in order to obtain high-quality histological preparations.

2.1 Preparation of the biopsy

Fixation in formol-saline, with subsequent paraffin-embedding, is of limited value in muscle biopsy pathology since it does not allow the use of enzyme histochemical or ultrastructural techniques. Formalin fixation is particularly appropriate to autopsy studies and as a means of

Table 2.1   Advantages and disadvantages of techniques of muscle biopsy

	Advantages	*Disadvantages*
Open surgical biopsy	1. Direct vision enables selection of tissue of sufficient quantity and of appropriate orientation. 2. Multiple samples obtainable through single incision. 3. Tissue for biochemical analysis obtained readily. 4. Coincidental skin biopsy possible. 5. Supravital studies of terminal innervation and end-plates possible by motor point biopsy. 6. No limitation on choice of muscle for biopsy. 7. Control of haemostasis.	1. Usually performed in operating theatre. 2. Incision and suture, with subsequent surgical scar. 3. Can only rarely be repeated. 4. Unsuitable for certain special applications, e.g. exercise physiology research. 5. Inexperienced surgeons tend to mishandle specimen, or distort it with intramuscular local anaesthetic injections.
Needle and conchotome biopsy	1. Does not require surgeon or operating theatre facilities. 2. No scar results. 3. Easily repeatable. 4. Special application in exercise physiology.	1. Poor control of haemostasis. 2. Limited choice of muscles for biopsy. 3. Small, randomly oriented specimen. 4. Metabolic and biochemical studies may be limited. 5. Rarely includes medium-sized blood vessels and muscle spindles.

conveniently storing material which can be used for study by conventional histological staining techniques. Thus stains for fibrous connective tissue, trichrome stains, and methods for calcium, RNA, DNA and glycogen, can be utilized. In addition, immunoperoxidase reactions can be applied. However, modern muscle histopathology depends primarily on a series of standardized enzyme histochemical reactions, applied to unfixed frozen tissue: without these, the diagnostic potential of the muscle biopsy is greatly restricted. Most of the classical histological techniques can be adapted for use in frozen tissue, and most modern enzyme histochemical reactions produce permanent results, so that the slides can be stored for future comparative study. Paraffin-embedded muscle is useful, nonetheless, in cytological studies of inflammatory cell

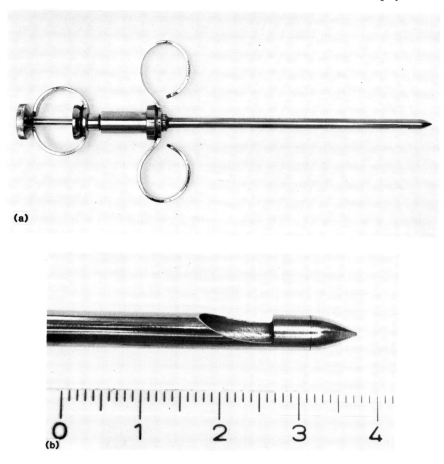

Fig. 2.1 (a) and (b) The modified Bergström needle (UCH needle) used for muscle biopsy to show the hollow cavity into which the biopsy is taken.

exudates, and of blood vessels. An immunohistochemical method, using an antineurofilament antibody, can be used to recognize Type 1 fibres in paraffin-embedded material (Oldfors and Seidal, 1989). Electron microscopy is applicable in certain diagnostic situations and it is useful to fix part of the biopsy for possible future study with the electron microscope, even if this material is not always processed fully.

The first step in preparation of the muscle biopsy is to select tissue for ultrastructural studies. Tiny cubes of tissue, no larger than 1 mm in any dimension, are cut from the biopsied muscle tissue and fixed for up to 4 h

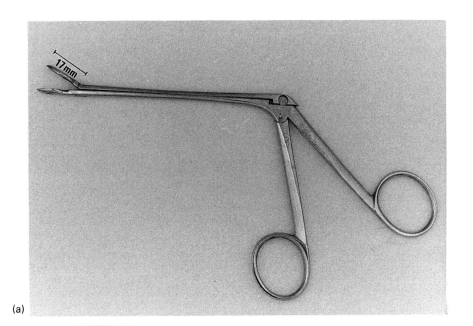

(a)

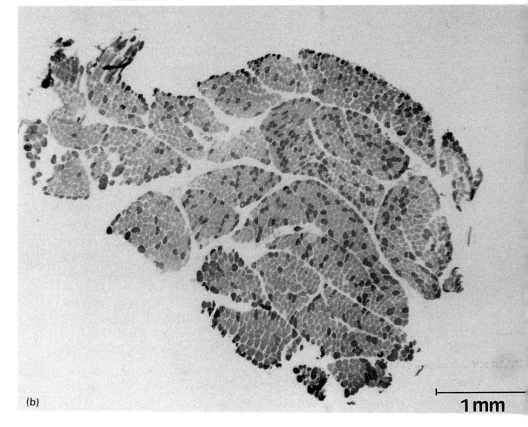

(b)

1mm

Table 2.2   Equipment used for snap-freezing muscle biopsies in the operating theatre, ward or outpatients department

---

Small open-topped vacuum flask half-filled with liquid nitrogen
Bottle of isopentane
Small metal drug container, suspended with stiff wire in the mouth of the flask
Long and short forceps
Scissors
Sharp, new, scalpel blades
Small cork discs (diameter 0.5 cm or less; thickness < 1 mm)
Tissue-Tek®
Small plastic containers suitable for storage of muscle specimens in liquid nitrogen or − 70°C refrigerator
Swabs
Ringer's solution
EM fixative (precooled to 4°C)
A few hypodermic needles (used for removing tissue from shaft of muscle biopsy needle)
A pair of asbestos gloves
Form for clinical details, etc.
Labels and pencil

---

in cooled glutaraldehyde or Karnovsky fixative. Routine plastic-embedding methods may then be followed, or the tissue may be stored for some time in buffer before embedding is carried out. It is important not to delay fixation of tissue for electron microscopy for more than a few minutes, in order to avoid swelling and disruption of mitochondria, and of the sarcoplasmic tubular system. In general, the smaller the tissue blocks taken into fixative, the better will be the results. It is usually quite easy to make sure that the blocks are cut at right angles to the orientation of the muscle fibres, so that true transverse and longitudinal sections can be prepared after embedding.

The remainder of the biopsy is snap-frozen for light microscopy. The materials needed for snap-freezing muscle are listed in Table 2.2. Isopentane is cooled in a small metal container suspended in the mouth of a vacuum flask of liquid nitrogen. Isopentane solidifies at this temperature (−160°C) and it is necessary to remove the isopentane container from the flask when the first solid-phase isopentane appears. The biopsy, moistened if necessary with buffered saline, or Ringer's

---

Fig. 2.2   (a) and (b) Conchotome (a), showing the muscle biopsy specimen (b) obtained by this technique; the specimen is larger than that obtained by needle biopsy. (Illustration kindly provided by Dr K.-G. Henriksson.)

solution, is cut cleanly with a sharp scalpel blade into small pieces no larger than 4 mm × 2 mm. The longer side of the specimen should be orientated longitudinally with the muscle fibres. Great care must be taken not to transfix the muscle specimen with a needle, or crush it with forceps or scissors, since this produces marked artefact.

Each piece of muscle tissue is mounted on a separate tiny, thin cork disc, previously prepared, using a small blob of Tissue-Tek® or other adhesive, and the cork disc and muscle tissue is then dropped lightly into

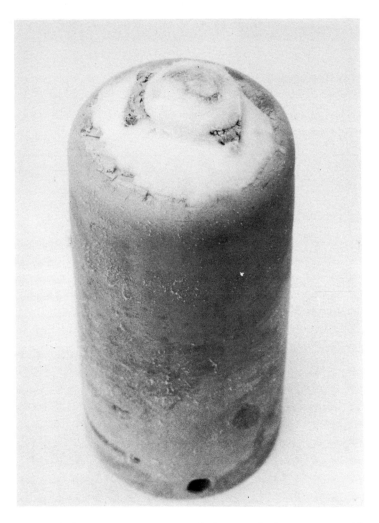

Fig. 2.3 Muscle biopsy specimen on cork disc, ready for sectioning. The cork layer, surrounded by ice, is frozen onto the precooled metal chuck.

the cooled isopentane. It is thus snap-frozen. It is usually possible to orientate the muscle tissue so that its fibres are arranged longitudinally or vertically on the cork disc. Transverse sections are more useful than longitudinal sections in diagnostic work, so most blocks should be arranged with the muscle fibres in the vertical plane. Occasionally, especially in biopsies taken from bipennate muscles, orientation is difficult and the muscle biopsy should then be taken, moistened with Ringer's solution, to a dissection stereomicroscope for proper orientation.

The frozen biopsy with its attached cork disc (Fig. 2.3) should be removed from the isopentane after a minute or so, placed into a previously cooled small plastic container (itself brought to the biopsy in liquid nitrogen) and then carried back to the laboratory immersed in the flask of liquid nitrogen itself. The specimen may then be stored in a refrigerator kept at $-70°C$ or in liquid nitrogen, in a special container. Specimens can be preserved indefinitely in liquid nitrogen without losing their enzyme reactivity and without fear of loss of material from mechanical or electrical failure in a refrigerator. It is thus not necessary to routinely process part of a biopsy into paraffin, after formalin fixation, for permanent storage. Furthermore, a small specimen is also available embedded in resin in the EM laboratory.

In some laboratories a freezing mixture of methanol and dry ice is used for cooling isopentane to an appropriate temperature for snap-freezing tissue. This method works well, although the freezing mixture is not at such a low temperature as when the liquid nitrogen method is used. This freezing mixture is cumbersome and so not easy to transport to the ward or operating theatre; we therefore prefer to use liquid nitrogen. It is possible to snap-freeze muscle biopsies directly in the flask of liquid nitrogen, by first coating the biopsy in talc before immersing it in the liquid nitrogen. The layer of talc helps to exclude air bubbles from the surface of the biopsy, thus facilitating rapid and uniform cooling of the muscle tissue. Failure to use talc means that a layer of air 'boils off' from the surface of the biopsy. This irregular heat flux from the biopsy causes artefact in the tissue, both from ice crystal formation within muscle fibres, and from cracking of the tissue. Finally, it is best to avoid trying to quench large muscle biopsies pinned to small matchsticks, or held in double Spencer Wells clamps, because these methods involve cooling large volumes of material of varying thermal conductivity and this frequently results in unacceptable ice crystal artefact.

2.2   Cutting sections

Sections of snap-frozen tissue are cut in a cryostat, at a temperature of about $-20°C$. Since the tissue is stored in liquid nitrogen at $-160°C$ there

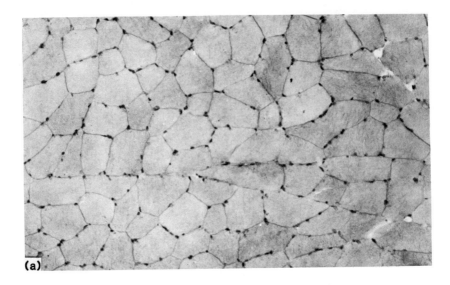

(a)

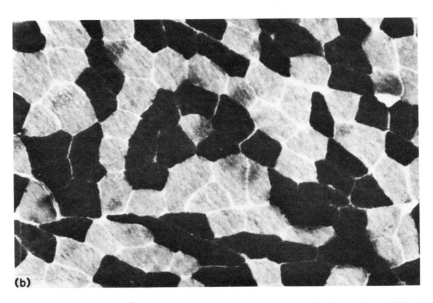

(b)

Fig. 2.4 Normal muscle in serial transverse section (Needle biopsy), × 140. (a) PAS. The polygonal muscle fibres are interdigitated, and the endomysial nuclei are subsarcolemmal. The different fibre types usually cannot be differentiated reliably in this technique; the fibres with the more marked glycogen content are Type 1 fibres. (b) ATPase, pH 9.4. In the alkali-stable ATPase reaction Type 2 fibres react darkly and Type 1 fibres appear pale. Note the Type 1 fibre surrounded by dark Type 2 fibres to the left of the centre of the illustration.

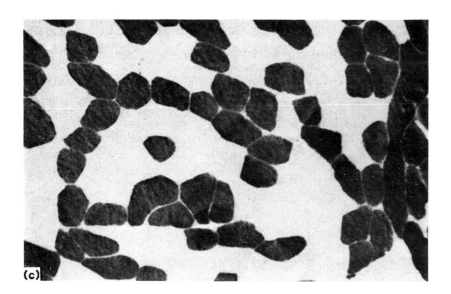

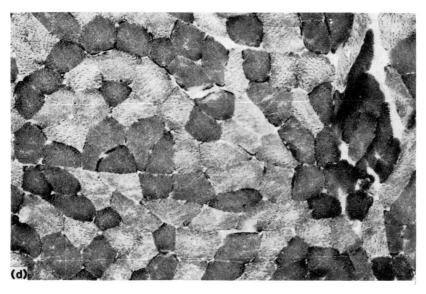

(c) ATPase, pH 4.3. This reaction is the converse of the result at pH 9.4. The pale fibre noted in (b) now reacts darkly, and its surrounding fibres are pale. (d) NADH. In this technique the granular intermyofibrillar material, including mitochondria, reacts darkly. Type 1 fibres, rich in mitochondria, appear dark, but fibres of both types react to some extent. The Type 2 fibres often show varying degrees of reactivity, but the subtypes cannot be consistently identified in this technique.

is a marked difference between the tissue and cryostat temperatures. The tissue block is fixed to a cooled chuck by a drop of water, which freezes the cork disc to the chuck; the cork insulates the biopsy itself from the relatively warm chuck, but the latter may itself be cooled to −160°C in liquid nitrogen and this manoeuvre helps to prevent ice crystals forming in the tissue. When the chuck has been fixed in the cryostat a little time should be allowed to elapse before sections are cut with a cooled knife.

A series of 6 to 12 transverse sections, each 5–8 μm thick, should be cut. It is sometimes useful to cut a similar series of longitudinal sections but most of the relevant information required for diagnosis can be obtained from transverse sections. A larger series of transverse sections may be required, particularly when the longitudinal extent of a particular abnormality is of importance. When the sections have been cut the cork disc and biopsy can be removed from the chuck by a sharp blow with a knife on the layer of ice between them, and the specimen can be returned to the liquid nitrogen tissue-storage container or refrigerator (−70°C) until it is required again.

2.3   Histological methods

A standard series of nine histological and enzyme histochemical methods (Fig. 2.4) should be carried out on each biopsy (Table 2.3). This series is intended to provide a basis for histopathological appraisal of the biopsy, to allow study of the distribution of different fibre types, and to identify a range of normal and abnormal structures within muscle fibres.

2.3.1   Haematoxylin and eosin (HE)

This well-known histological stain is the most useful of all the techniques used in muscle biopsy work. In cryostat sections the muscle fibres are free

Table 2.3   Routine series of histological methods for muscle biopsies (nine sections)

Haematoxylin and eosin (HE)
Nicotine adenine dinucleotide dehydrogenase tetrazolium reductase (NADH)
Myosin adenosine triphosphatase (ATPase) – preincubated at pH 9.4, 4.6 and 4.3, respectively
Modified Gomori trichrome
Periodic acid Schiff (PAS)
Oil red O/Ehrlich's haematoxylin
Verhoeff van Gieson

of fixation artefact and thus appear as slightly rounded structures, neatly interdigitating with each other and with their endomysial capillaries (Fig. 2.4). Abnormal variation in fibre size, fibres which have lost their normal granularity, basophilic regenerating fibres, necrotic fibres and small pyknotic fibres can all easily be recognized. Any inflammatory cell response can be identified, in relation to muscle fibres, interstitial tissue or blood vessels. Nerve fibres can also be studied within muscle biopsies in HE stains. Rare abnormalities, such as granulomas, parasites or tumour deposits, are also best seen in the HE preparation. However, fat cells and fibrous tissues are not well delineated.

2.3.2   Reduced nicotine adenine dinucleotide tetrazolium reductase (NADH)

This oxidative enzyme reaction identifies mitochondria which contain the cell's oxidative enzymes, but there is also a less specific reaction with sarcoplasmic tubules. Since both mitochondria and sarcoplasmic tubules are located between the myofibrils this enzyme reaction delineates the intermyofibrillar anatomy of the muscle fibres. The reaction product is seen as a coarsely granular or reticulate deposition throughout the fibre, except in zones occupied by subsarcolemmal nuclei. Two fibre types can be recognized by the density of the reaction but in most muscles a large number of fibres with an intermediate reaction occur (Fig. 2.4). Fibres with a strong reaction represent fibres dependent on oxidative metabolism, the slow-twitch Type 1 fibres. Less strongly reactive fibres are capable of anaerobic, glycolytic metabolism; these are the fast-twitch Type 2 fibres (Table 2.4). Sections prepared for NADH tend to lift off glass slides, thus making microscopy at higher magnifications difficult. This can be prevented by partially fixing the dried section on the slide with 70% alcohol before starting the enzyme reaction.

Succinic dehydrogenase (SDH) may also be identified by an enzyme histochemical technique. This reaction is specific for SDH and thus for mitochondria, a useful method when a mitochondrial myopathy is suspected.

2.3.3   Myosin ATPase methods

Fibre typing is usually carried out, by convention, on myosin ATPase preparations (Table 2.4). The currently used classification of fibre types in man was devised in myosin ATPase preparations preincubated at pH 9.4, 4.6 and 4.3 (Brooke and Kaiser, 1970). Other classifications of fibre types, based on different histochemical techniques, have been devised but these are complex and less precise for clinical pathology (Romanul, 1964). With preincubation at pH 9.4 two fibre types can be differentiated, darkly

Table 2.4 Classification of muscle fibre types in standard histological methods (from Swash and Schwartz, 1988)

	Type 1	Type 2A	Type 2B	Type 2C
Myosin ATPase				
pH 9.4	Pale	Dark	Dark	Dark
pH 4.6	Dark	Pale	Dark	Dark
pH 4.3	Dark	Pale	Pale	Intermediate
NADH	Dark	Intermediate	Intermediate	Intermediate
PAS	Pale	Dark	Intermediate	Intermediate
Oil red O				
(lipid droplets)	Plentiful	Sparse	Sparse	Sparse
Myophosphorylase	Pale	Dark	Dark	Dark
HE	Darker red	Red	Red	Red
Physiological characteristics	Slow twitch	Fast twitch: Fatigue-resistant	Fast twitch: Rapidly fatiguing	—

reacting Type 2 fibres and lightly reacting Type 1 fibres. This reaction is reversed in the preincubation at pH 4.3. In intermediate preincubations, usually carried out at pH 4.6, three fibre types can be recognized, consisting of Type 1, Type 2A and Type 2B fibres (Table 2.4). At this pH, Type 1 and Type 2B fibres are both dark; the Type 1 fibres are usually darker than the Type 2B fibres (Fig. 2.4). In the myosin ATPase reaction, myofibrils react positively; this reaction thus demonstrates the myofibrillar material itself. The distribution and packing density of myofibrils may thus be assessed by this method. Type 2C fibres probably represent precursors of all the other fibres. They comprise 20% of fibres in newborns but only about 1% in adult muscle (Colling-Saltin, 1978). The availability of an antineurofilament antibody that recognizes Type 1 muscle fibres in paraffin-embedded muscle (Oldfors and Seidal, 1989) will allow the detection of changes in the pattern of innervation in stored tissue.

2.3.4   *Periodic acid Schiff method (PAS)*

This technique is used to demonstrate glycogen, and membranous structures containing mucopolysaccharide, glycoproteins, mucoprotein, glycolipids and phospholipids (Fig. 2.4). The presence of glycogen can be established by incubating a second section after predigestion with diastase; any remaining reaction product must then be due to cellular or tubular membranes. The PAS method does not produce a reaction which can easily be quantified, but generally two fibre types can be recognized (Table 2.4) and any increase in the glycogen content of muscle fibres can be established. The technique is best carried out after alcohol prefixation of the dried section, which prevents washing-out of glycogen during the preparative procedure. The method may also be combined with a haematoxylin or other nuclear counterstain, which aids identification of individual fibres in the serial sections.

2.3.5   Modified Gomori trichrome

This trichrome method, modified for use in cryostat sections, has become deservedly popular in muscle biopsies. Muscle fibres stain greenish-blue, the intermyofibrillar tubules, mitochondria and membrane-bound fat droplets appear a bright red and the endomysial connective/fibrous tissue stains green. Nuclei appear reddish-brown and are thus easily seen. The popularity of this stain derives from the ease with which necrotic or hyaline fibres can be seen, and abnormal intrasarcoplasmic inclusions, such as rod bodies, and abnormalities of mitochondria or of the sarcoplasmic tubular system can also be recognized. The presence of these abnormalities can be confirmed by electron microscopy.

In well-prepared Gomori-stained sections two fibre types can be recognized by their differential sarcoplasmic staining, just as in well-stained HE preparations. The method depends very much on good histological techniques; dried sections, too thick sections, or stale Gomori stain will all lead to poor results, often with areas of blotchy pink pigment across the section.

2.3.6   Oil red O/Ehrlich's haematoxylin

Neutral lipids can be demonstrated by several methods including oil red O and Sudan black. The oil red O technique produces a bright red reaction which is easily seen as small red droplets in the fibres. The Type 1 fibres contain larger and more numerous lipid droplets than the Type 2 fibres. A haematoxylin counterstain is useful because not only does it indicate the position of the muscle fibre nuclei (Fig. 2.4), but it picks out basophilic regenerating fibres particularly clearly. In some myopathies lipid droplets accumulate, as in carnitine deficiency and in steroid myopathy.

2.3.7   Verhoeff van Gieson stain

Fibrous tissue appears red in this method and this is sometimes a useful technique for the assessment of increased interstitial fibrous tissue in myopathies. Similar delineation of fibrous tissue can be made with the

Gomori method, but the Verhoeff van Gieson is easier to carry out satisfactorily. It may also be usefully combined with Hart's method for elastic tissue.

2.3.8   Other histological techniques

A number of other techniques are sometimes useful in diagnosis, particularly when specific problems arise. For example, the myo-phosphorylase technique, formerly used for muscle fibre typing, is useful when McArdle's disease (myophosphorylase deficiency) is suspected. It is often helpful to use specific histological methods for intrasarcoplasmic RNA and DNA. Methods are also available for intracellular calcium deposition and such as von Kossa's method and alizarin red. Immunoperoxidase methods for demonstration of serum immunoproteins in muscle fibres or in inflammatory cells, or of immune complexes in blood vessels, are occasionally of value. Specific monoclonal antibody methods for demonstrating cell surface markers have been used in identifying B cells, T cells and their subtypes in inflammatory myopathies. A monoclonal antibody raised against dystrophin is capable of demonstrating the underlying abnormality in X-linked Duchenne and related muscular dystrophies. Some of these methods, suitable for cryostat sections, are listed in Table 2.5.

2.3.9   Plastic-embedded material

Semithin sections of plastic- or resin-embedded muscle are of great value (Fig. 2.5). Indeed, in many instances almost as much information may be gained from study of semithin sections as may be obtained from electron microscopy itself, especially if high magnifications or phase-contrast microscopy are used. In most laboratories toluidine blue stains are used, but other methods are available. Inclusions within muscle fibres, or abnormalities of subcellular organelles such as tubules, or mitochondria, can often be recognized in these semithin sections.

2.3.10   Electron microscopy

Transmission electron microscopy was used to formulate modern concepts of the subcellular organization of muscle fibres, and the structure of the sliding filaments responsible for muscular contraction (Fig. 2.5). However, the advent of enzyme histochemistry and of toluidine blue staining of semithin sections has made electron microscopy less useful in routine diagnosis of muscle biopsies than might at first be supposed. The main value of ultrastructural studies by transmission

Table 2.5 Special histological techniques applicable to cryostat sections of muscle

Method	Indication
Toluidine blue	A quick method, comparable to HE as a screening stain. It may also be used to demonstrate metachromasia
Acid phosphatase	Demonstrating autophagic vacuoles in degenerating and many regenerating muscle fibres
Acridine orange	A fluorescence method specific for RNA
Methylgreen pyronin	Demonstrates RNA (red) and DNA (green). Increased sarcoplasmic RNA is an indication of protein synthesis, and thus muscle fibre regeneration. Increased sarcoplasmic DNA is found in degenerating or necrotic fibres
Myophosphorylase	(See Table 2.4.) Prominent in Type 2 fibres. The enzyme is absent in McArdle's disease
Phosphofructokinase	Deficiency of this enzyme occurs rarely in a syndrome similar to McArdle's disease
Cytochrome oxidase	Mitochondria-specific enzyme, useful in mitochondrial cytopathies
Myoadenylate deaminase	Type 2 fibre cytosol enzyme that is deficient in some patients with fatigue
Von Kossa or alizarin red	Calcium
Acetylcholinesterase with or without silver impregnation	Useful for demonstrating motor end-plates
Non-specific esterase	Increased in denervated fibres
Immunoperoxidase methods	For immunoproteins. These methods are generally not useful in routine diagnosis

electron microscopy is thus as a research technique. Generally, transmission electron microscopy cannot be expected to provide diagnostic information if no abnormality is discerned in light microscopy. Ultrastructural studies have proven to be most useful in the investigation of the congenital or benign myopathies of childhood, in which specific abnormalities of diagnostic value may occur, and in mitochondrial cytopathies, in which characteristic abnormalities in mitochondrial morphology are found. In addition, ultrastructural studies are useful in characterizing the morphology of inclusion bodies in muscle fibres in certain inherited myopathies, and in studying vacuolar myopathies,

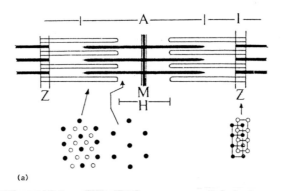

(a)

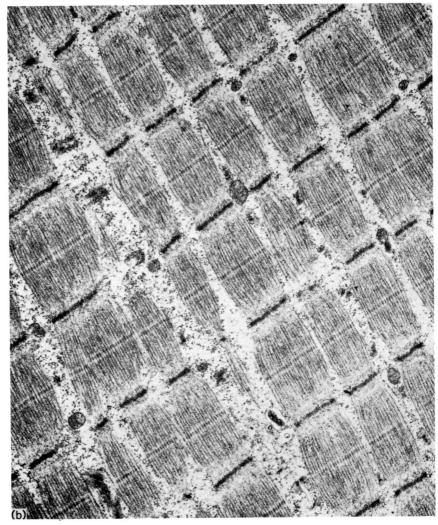

(b)

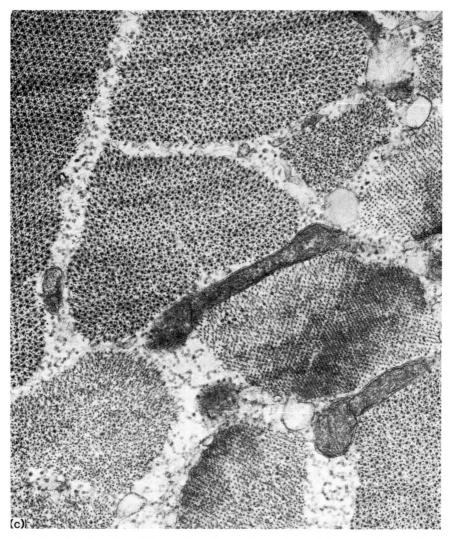

Fig. 2.5 (a) Drawing of the sliding filament structure of the myofilament in longitudinal and transverse planes. Compare with the ultrastructural appearance in the longitudinal ($\times$ 18 000) (b) and transverse ($\times$ 46 800) electron micrographs (c). (After Landon, 1982.)

particularly in differentiating lysosomal vacuoles from other vacuolar changes, e.g. dilated T tubules. Satellite cells proliferate at the onset of regeneration and can best be recognized by electron microscopy. Motor end-plates are sometimes available for study in ultrathin sections but diagnostically specific changes are rarely seen in these structures.

Freeze-fracture electron microscopy has been used in research on membrane structure in the muscular dystrophies, especially in Duchenne muscular dystrophy, and scanning electron microscopy may have a similar application. Neither of these techniques has, as yet, revealed abnormalities sufficiently specific to be used in clinical diagnosis.

2.3.11   Autopsy methods

Muscle obtained at autopsy is generally suitable for study by most of the histological and enzyme histological methods discussed above, provided that specimens comparable in size to those obtained at muscle biopsy are prepared by snap-freezing in isopentane cooled with liquid nitrogen. Most muscle enzymes can be demonstrated in autopsy specimens even as long as 48 h after death, particularly if the cadaver has been kept adequately cooled in a refrigerator. It is particularly important to prepare muscle specimens with these techniques at autopsy in order to study the distribution of abnormality in neuromuscular diseases and this has, so far, been much neglected in muscle pathology. Many neuromuscular diseases are still defined only in terms of their muscle biopsy appearances. Autopsies of patients dying with neuromuscular diseases should not therefore be restricted to the examination of a few proximal muscles, for example biceps brachii and quadriceps femoris, using only formalin-fixed, paraffin-embedded material. Instead, a wide selection of bulbar, and of proximal and distal, upper and lower limb, muscles should be studied in cryostat sections. Normal material has been investigated by Polgar et al. (1973) and by Johnson et al. (1973), who studied 36 different muscles at autopsy. Cryostat sections have considerable advantages over paraffin sections. Not only may enzyme reactions be utilized but the morphology of individual fibres is more easily studied. Paraffin sections of muscle, even at autopsy, are prone to be marred by artefact from shrinkage, cracking and even from imperfect fixation.

Attempts to examine autopsied muscle samples by electron microscopy, however, produce unsatisfactory results because of post-mortem autolysis.

2.4   Histological techniques for other structures found in muscle

Muscle biopsies often contain small nerve fibre bundles and, less commonly, other structures, such as motor end-plates, muscle spindles, Golgi tendon organs and Pacinian corpuscles may be present. These may not be easily identified at first, but it is important to recognize them as normal structures in sections of muscle. Sometimes, abnormalities may be recognized in these structures.

2.4.1   Nerve fibre bundles

These can be recognized in HE preparations by the characteristic bluish-red colour of myelin (Fig. 2.6). Silver impregnations such as Schofield's technique for frozen sections or the Glees and Marsland method for paraffin-embedded tissue may be useful. Most nerve fibre bundles are found in interfascicular planes.

2.4.2   Motor end-plates

Motor end-plates are not frequently found in muscle biopsies since most biopsies are taken away from the motor point. They are difficult to recognize in HE (Fig. 2.7) or van Gieson stains and are not visualized in the routine enzyme preparations, but the acetylcholinesterase method demonstrates the end-plate apparatus in sectioned material, and a modification of this technique, described by Pestronk and Drachman (1979), enables it to be combined with silver impregnation in frozen material. Another technique, used for studies of motor end-plates in man, uses supravital methylene blue, injected into the muscle at the time of the biopsy (Fig. 2.8). This method can produce impregnations not only of the terminal nerve tree and preterminal axonal sprouts of the motor end-plates, but also of intramuscular nerve fibres.

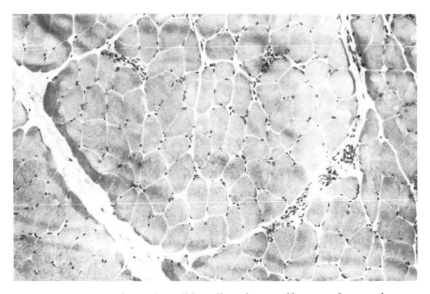

Fig. 2.6   × 140; HE. Several small bundles of nerve fibres can be seen between and within fasciculi.

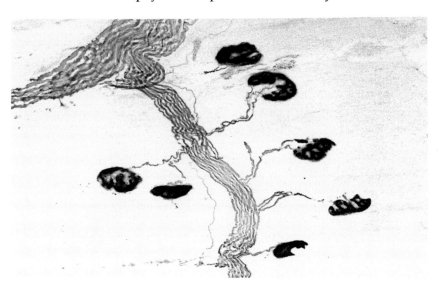

Fig. 2.7 Motor end-plates. Pestronk and Drachman silver/cholinesterase method. × 132. The end-plate morphology with its terminal innervation is displayed in this method. (Illustration kindly provided by Professor L. Duchen.)

At autopsy the acetylcholinesterase method may be used up to 48 h or so after death. Paraffin-embedded or frozen sections can be used for silver impregnations and block impregnation methods in fresh muscle have also been utilized (Swash and Fox, 1972).

2.4.3 Other intramuscular organelles

Muscle spindles are sometimes found in muscle biopsies, particularly in open biopsies (see Fig. 1.2). Special techniques are available for studying the innervation of these complex sensory receptors (see Swash and Fox, 1972).

2.4.4 Other studies on muscle biopsies

A number of quantitative biochemical assays of muscle enzyme activity, for example in suspected glycogen storage disorders, have been used for diagnosis, and similar techniques have recently been applied to patients with mitochondrial myopathies in order to define the underlying mitochondrial metabolic disorder (Morgan-Hughes, 1986).

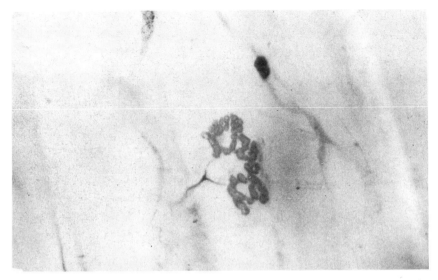

Fig. 2.8 Methylene blue preparation. Normal rat motor end-plate. Note the preterminal axonal branching and the subneural, presynaptic apparatus.

2.4.5 Artefacts

A number of artefacts occur both in frozen and paraffin-embedded muscle. In frozen muscle the most common artefact is due to ice crystal formation, which produces a speckled pattern of small holes in the muscle fibres (Fig. 2.9). These usually have sharply defined, rather concave borders, with sharp corners, but they can be confused with lipid droplets. When severe they may mar interpretation of the biopsy. They may be avoided by scrupulous attention to snap-freezing technique and especially by care during section cutting. They are particularly likely to occur if the knife blade or the slides are warmer than the temperature of the muscle tissue. If a block is affected by ice crystal artefact, the sections can sometimes be improved by allowing the block to melt to room temperature, and then refreezing it. However, this often results in slight swelling of the fibres, shown by a rounded appearance.

Knife-cutting artefacts, consisting of ridges of variable thickness in the section, are fairly common and are usually due to vibration in the cryostat. Blunt knives may cause a similar abnormality, or lead to tears in the section. Folded sections, especially at one edge, usually result from poor technique during the enzyme or staining reactions. If a block is allowed to dry before snap-freezing, the fibres at its edge become shrunken, vitreous and excessively eosinophilic, an appearance which

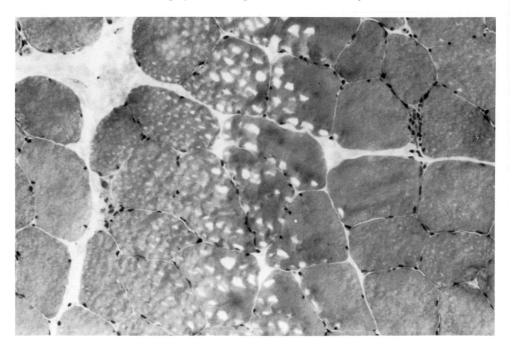

Fig. 2.9   × 380; HE. Ice crystal artefact. This artefact is often found in only part of a section – it may then result from differential warming or cooling in different parts of the section, during section cutting, or when fixing the block to the chuck in the cryostat.

may easily be confused with the hypercontracted, hyalinized fibres found in Duchenne muscular dystrophy. Haemorrhage, displacing fibres in a fascicle, is invariably due to surgical trauma. Similarly, apparent oedematous displacement of fibres from each other in a fascicle may be due to local anaesthetic inadvertently injected into the muscle at the biopsy site.

Muscle biopsies prepared for paraffin sections are vulnerable to fixation artefact, in which muscle fibres undergo abrupt hypercontraction with loss of cross-striations and loss of orientation. This can be avoided by pre-preparation in Ringer's solution for 15–30 min before fixation in buffered formol saline. Formalin-fixation of biopsied or autopsied muscle is best accomplished by pinning short narrow strips of muscle on to a card, in a slightly stretched state. Fixation should not be prolonged longer than a few hours or overnight if the best histological results are to be obtained. Paraffin-embedding should be carried out using a slow embedding schedule.

Muscle prepared for electron microscopy is also vulnerable to artefact (Mair and Tomé, 1972). Fixation should be accomplished as rapidly as possible after removal of tissue from the patient in order to avoid mitochondrial swelling. It should not be prolonged longer than about 4 h, the muscle then being best stored in buffered saline prior to plastic-embedding.

References

Brooke, M.H. and Kaiser, K.K. (1970) Muscle fiber types: how many and what kind? *Arch. Neurol.*, **23**, 369–379.

Colling-Saltin, A. (1978) Enzyme histochemistry on skeletal muscle of the human foetus. *J. Neurol. Sci.*, **39**, 169–185.

Edwards, R.H.T. (1971) Percutaneous needle-biopsy of skeletal muscle in diagnosis and research. *Lancet*, **2**, 593–596.

Henriksson, K.-G. (1979) Semi-open muscle biopsy technique: a simple outpatient procedure. *Acta Neurol. Scand.*, **59**, 317–323.

Johnson, M.A., Polgar, J., Weightman, D. and Appleton, D. (1973) Data on the distribution of fibre types in thirty-six human muscles: an autopsy study. *J. Neurol. Sci.*, **18**, 111–129.

Landon, D.N. (1982) Skeletal muscle: normal morphology, development and innervation. In *Skeletal Muscle Pathology* (eds F.L. Mastaglia and J.N. Walton), Churchill Livingstone, Edinburgh, ch. 1, p. 187.

Mair, W.G.P. and Tomé, F.M.S. (1972) *Atlas of the Ultrastructure of Diseased Human Muscle*, Churchill Livingstone, Edinburgh.

Morgan-Hughes, J.A. (1986) The mitochondrial myopathies. In *Myology* vol 2 (eds A.G. Engel and B.Q. Banker), McGraw-Hill, New York, pp. 1709–1743.

Oldfors, A. and Seidal, T. (1989) Immunohistochemical demonstration of different muscle fibre types in paraffin sections. *Histopathology*, **15**, 420–423.

Pestronk, A. and Drachman, D.B. (1979) A new stain for quantitative measurement of sprouting at neuromuscular junctions. *Muscle Nerve*, **1**, 70–74.

Polgar, J., Johnson, M.A., Weightman, D. and Appleton, D. (1973) Data on fibre size in thirty-six human muscles: an autopsy study. *J. Neurol. Sci.*, **19**, 307–318.

Romanul, F.C. (1964) Enzymes in muscle. I. Histochemical studies of enzymes in individual muscle fibers. *Arch. Neurol.*, **11**, 355–358.

Swash, M. and Fox, K.P. (1972) Techniques for the demonstration of human muscle spindle innervation in neuromuscular disease. *J. Neurol. Sci.*, **15**, 291–302.

Swash, M. and Schwartz, M.S. (1988) *Neuromuscular Diseases: A Practical Approach to Diagnosis and Management*, 2nd edn, Springer-Verlag, London, pp. 456.

3   Histological and morphometric characteristics of normal muscle

Muscle fibres in frozen sections, prepared as discussed in Chapter 2, normally take the form of irregular polygons with slightly rounded sides, arranged in close apposition. In an idealized cross-section of normal muscle, if all muscle fibres were of equal size each fibre would conform to a hexagonal shape (Fig. 3.1), but Type 1, Type 2A and Type 2B fibres differ somewhat in their mean diameter and so there is variation not only in size, but in shape. In addition to the *histological appearance* of muscle fibres and of the endomysial and interfascicular tissue and organelles, the size of fibres, the *distribution of fibres* of different histochemical types and the relative *predominance* of different fibre types can be studied.

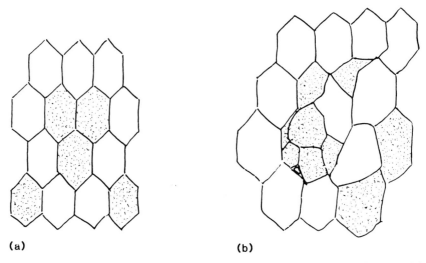

(a)   (b)

Fig. 3.1   If all muscle fibres were hexagonal (a) and of equal size, they would interdigitate in a regular pattern, but not all fibres conform to this shape. Fibres smaller than normal, or fibres with fewer 'sides', alter the pattern of interdigitation (b).

3.1   Fibre size

Muscle fibre size has usually been expressed as the lesser transverse diameter (Brooke and Engel, 1969), since this measurement is least affected by variations in the plane of section of the muscle fibre away from the true transverse plane. Fibre diameters can be measured simply with an eye-piece micrometer calibrated against a graduated scale, or from photographic enlargements of transverse sections of muscle. Care must be taken either to measure *all* the fibres in a biopsy, however large or small, or to measure *all* the fibres contained within an arbitrary number, not less than 5, of different microscope fields, selected randomly in the biopsy. At least 100 fibres of each type should be measured. Sufficient fibres are usually available in needle muscle biopsies for these quantitative studies.

Fibre size increases with maturation (Fig. 3.2). At one year of age the mean fibre diameter is 16 μm and at age 10 years, 40 μm. It increases by 2 μm for each year to age 5 years and then by 3 μm for each year to age 9 years. Adult diameters are achieved between age 12 and 15 years (Table 3.1). In adult men most muscle fibres are within the range 40–80 μm diameter, and in adult women 30–70 μm. Fibres smaller than 20 μm, or larger than 100 μm, diameter are not usually found in muscle. In childhood, Type 1 and Type 2 fibres are of similar size to each other. In adult women Type 1 fibres are larger than Type 2 fibres, but in men the reverse obtains. In normal subjects muscle fibre diameters have been thoroughly studied in the biceps brachii, lateral quadriceps and deltoid muscles (Table 3.1). Polgar *et al.* (1973) measured the mean diameters of Type 1 and Type 2 fibres in an autopsy study of 36 different human muscles in six male subjects. This study showed that Type 2 fibres were of larger diameter than Type 1 fibres in 90% of the muscles examined, but that this difference in mean diameter was usually not statistically significant. Both fibre types were equally variable in fibre size, with moderately large ranges of diameter values in individual subjects. In some muscles, the muscle fibres were larger in deep than in superficial samples (Lexell and Taylor, 1989). Blomstrand and Ekblom (1982) have shown that there is only a very small variation in fibre size and distribution indices in normal subjects subjected to repeated biopsies of the quadriceps (vastus lateralis) muscle. Further, using area measurements, they noted that there was concordance between the two legs in individual subjects (Blomstrand *et al.*, 1984).

The standard deviation of the mean fibre diameter in normal muscle is usually less than 10 μm. Another quantitative method for expressing variability in fibre diameter, suggested by Brooke and Engel (1969), uses weighting factors to indicate the presence of fibres larger or smaller than

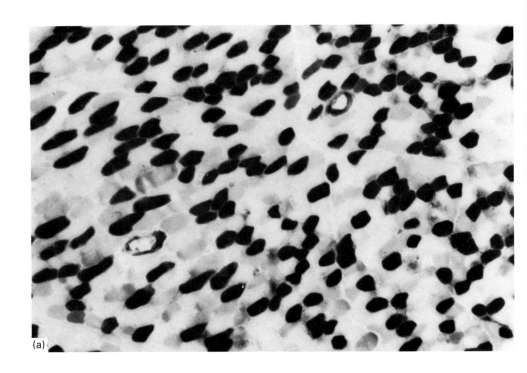

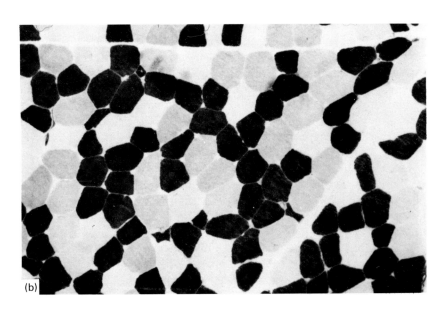

Table 3.1 Normal mean muscle fibre diameters in adult biceps brachii (μm) from Brooke and Engel (1969)

	Type 1	Type 2
Men	64	73
Women	57	47

those within the normal range; that is 40–80 μm in adult men and 30–70 μm in adult women. This method gives increased numerical weight to very large or to very small fibres, the result being expressed as hypertrophy factors or atrophy factors. Thus, in men fibres of 30–40 μm diameter are given a weight of 1 and fibres of 10–20 μm diameter a weight of 3. These weights are divided by the total number of fibres measured. The resulting number is multiplied by 1000 to produce an atrophy factor. A similar method is used to calculate the hypertrophy factor in the same muscle fibres.

A simpler method of showing fibre atrophy or hypertrophy is to construct fibre-size histograms, expressed as a percentage of the total number of fibres measured. This histogram can be compared visually, or by subtraction, with normal muscle biopsies from the same muscles.

Computer-assisted methods of planimetry for measuring fibre area are also available (Standstedt *et al.*, 1982); these usually involve the observer in tracing the outline of muscle fibres onto a graphics tablet linked to a microcomputer, using a photomicrograph or a drawing tube attached to the microscope (Mahon *et al.*, 1984). The value of these measurements in relation to fibre diameter measurements remains to be established (see Slavin *et al.*, 1982). All these methods are time consuming and rarely contribute to diagnosis, although they are useful in research, for example in studies of disuse atrophy or exercise-induced hypertrophy of muscle fibres. Automatic methods are available, but these always require manual checking and correction.

Fig. 3.2 (a) Infant muscle (aged 2 years). × 237; ATPase, pH 4.6. The three fibre types are well developed, but the muscle fibres are very much smaller than in the adult. The fascicular pattern can be clearly seen.
(b) Adult muscle × 140; ATPase, pH 4.6. There is a mosaic distribution of Type 1 (dark), Type 2A (pale) and Type 2B (intermediate) fibres, with approximately equal numbers of fibres of each type. This muscle is normal, apart from the presence of a few, isolated, small Type 1 fibres. The interfascicular planes can be clearly recognized.

3.2   Fibre-type distribution

Muscle fibres are distributed in a mosaic pattern of the different fibre types, the mosaic approximately conforming to a random distribution. The muscle fibres making up individual motor units are distributed over a wide cross-sectional area of any muscle, so that individual muscle fibres in a motor unit are located in many different fascicles (see Fig. 1.1). It is unusual for more than two or three muscle fibres within a motor unit to be in contact with each other (Edstrom and Kugelberg, 1968); most such fibres are not situated in apposition with each other in normal muscle. Statistical analysis suggests that groups of six fibres are unlikely to occur in normal muscle, so that enclosed fibres, i.e. fibres surrounded by fibres of the same histochemical type, are not found in normal muscle (Willison, 1980). The mosaic pattern of normal muscle thus consists of many different intermingled motor units each made up of fibres of one of the three major histochemical types. However, this relationship depends to some extent on the relative predominance of a particular fibre type within a muscle. For example the soleus muscle contains predominantly Type 1 fibres and in this muscle the Type 1 fibres therefore often appear close to each other. This is particularly prominent when 70% or more fibre-type predominance is present. In most muscles Type 2 fibres predominate; in the most commonly biopsied muscles, the biceps brachii, deltoid and quadriceps, there are twice as many Type 2 as Type 1 fibres. However, in these muscles there are similar proportions of Type 2A, Type 2B and Type 1 muscle fibres.

The relative predominance of the different fibre types is, to some extent, an inherited characteristic. Some people tend to have more Type 1 fibres than others (Komi *et al.*, 1977), a characteristic likely to lead to particular abilities in endurance athletic events. Training does not influence fibre-type predominance or distribution (Salmons and Henriksson, 1981). Endurance training increases the number of capillaries surrounding individual muscle fibres (Andersson and Henriksson, 1977), and may increase the proportion of Type 2A fibres (Edstrom and Grimby, 1986). Disuse tends to reverse the effects of training. In weight-lifters trained for sudden maximal contraction of muscles Type 2B fibres may show selective hypertrophy (Saltin *et al.*, 1976).

3.3   Fibre-type predominance

In normal muscle Type 1 muscle fibres constitute less than 55% of the fibres in a biopsy (Fig. 2.4), and Type 2 muscle fibres less than 80% (Dubowitz, 1985). Predominance of Type 1 or Type 2 fibres is thus said to occur if these figures (Fig. 3.3) are exceeded (see Chapter 4).

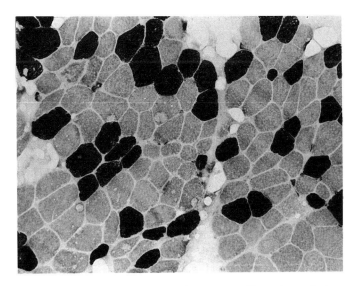

Fig. 3.3   ATPase pH 4.3. Fibre-type predominance. There is a relative excess of Type 2 fibres (80%). The biopsy was taken from the quadriceps muscle of a patient with a slowly progressive limb-girdle dystrophy.

3.4   Histological features

Several other features of normal muscle can be quantified and these are useful measures of normality.

3.4.1   Central nucleation

In transverse section each muscle fibre contains one or more subsarco-lemmal nuclei. Normal muscle fibres contain less than 8 such nuclei (Greenfield *et al.*, 1957). Centrally located nuclei are found in less than 3% of normal muscle fibres (Greenfield *et al.*, 1957).

3.4.2   Fat and fibrous tissue

The interfascicular planes of normal muscle consist of connective and fibrous tissue, but in most biopsies this plane of tissue is thin. Most muscles also contain thick fibrous planes acting as internal tendons or sites of insertion of muscle fibres but these should not normally be included in a biopsy. The larger interfascicular boundaries may contain some fatty tissue but this is an uncommon feature of normal muscle, and fatty tissue does not infiltrate or replace muscle fibres themselves in normal biopsies. These connective tissue septa contain elastic tissue.

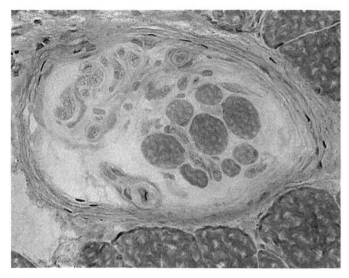

(a)

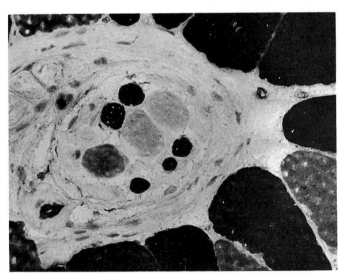

(b)

Fig. 3.4 Muscle spindle in transverse section. × 560. (a) Gomori trichrome. The spindle capsule, periaxial space and intrafusal muscle fibres can be seen. These fibres are much smaller than the extrafusal skeletal muscle fibres themselves.
(b) ATPase, pH 4.6. There are three histochemical types of intrafusal muscle fibre in this reaction; darkly reactive, small nuclear chain fibres; and intermediate, and lightly reactive nuclear bag fibres. The capsule is virtually non-reactive. It is important to recognize that these isolated small muscle fibres are normal structures. The extrafusal fibres show ice crystal artefact.

The endomysium is thin and barely discernible in young people, but thickens slightly with increasing age (Rubinstein, 1960; Swash and Fox, 1972a). This endomysial tissue is not normally thick enough to cause more than very slight separation of muscle fibres from each other.

3.4.3 Fibre splitting

In normal muscle, fibre splitting is found only at the tendinous insertion of muscle fibres (Bell and Conen, 1968). This can be recognized by the proximity of these split fibres to bands of collagenous tissue. Fibre splitting may also occur in normal subjects following training, when it represents a response accompanying work-induced hypertrophy (Edgerton, 1970; Hall-Craggs, 1970). Regenerating and necrotic fibres are not found in normal muscle.

3.4.4 Muscle spindles

Muscle spindles occur in all human skeletal muscles except the facial muscles and the diaphragm (Fig. 3.4). The fibrous capsule of the spindle encloses 4–14 intrafusal muscle fibres in a mucopolysaccharide-filled periaxial space (Swash and Fox, 1972a). These intrafusal muscle fibres are smaller than adult extrafusal muscle fibres but larger than the extrafusal muscle fibres of infants. The intrafusal muscle fibres have complex enzyme histochemical reactions, which differ in the two main types of fibre, the larger nuclear bag and the smaller nuclear chain fibres (for review see Swash, 1990). Spindles are more frequently found in motor point biopsies than at other sites in individual muscles. Most spindles occur close to neurovascular bundles in the interfascicular plane.

Golgi tendon organs occur in tendinous septa; they are rarely found in muscle biopsies. Occasionally Pacinian corpuscles are seen in muscle, usually in close relation to muscle spindles.

Muscle spindles and Golgi tendon organs can be recognized in transverse or longitudinal sections of muscle, either at biopsy or at autopsy. At autopsy gold chloride or silver nitrate block impregnation techniques have been used to demonstrate the innervation of muscle spindles in whole mounts (Fig. 3.5), but this is a specialized technique requiring microdissection or teasing using a stereo microscope (Swash and Fox, 1972b).

3.4.5 Nerves

Small nerve bundles are almost always seen in open muscle biopsies, and frequently in needle biopsies. They are found in the perifascicular regions

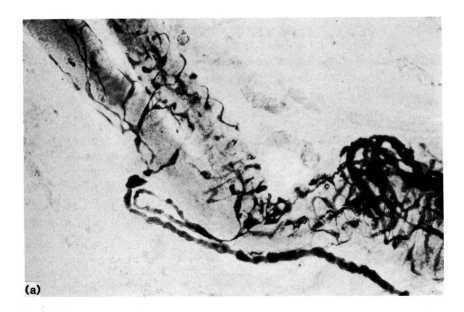

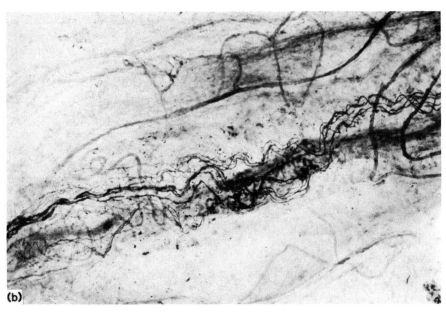

Fig. 3.5 (a) Muscle spindle × 350. Teased Barker and Ip silver impregnation to demonstrate the pattern of sensory innervation in a de-efferented baboon spindle. The primary sensory ending is to the right, and the secondary to the left of the illustration. (b) Muscle spindle × 140. Teased Barker and Ip silver impregnation. The motor and sensory nerve fibres in this human spindle form a

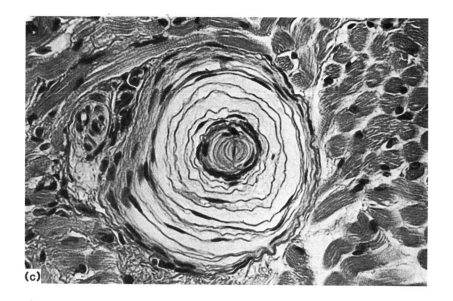

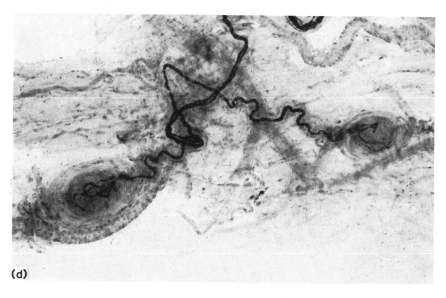

complex distribution of endings on the intrafusal muscle fibres. Note the capillaries running across the microscope field. The thicker sensory nerve fibres and the fine gamma efferent (motor) fibres can be recognized. (c) Pacinian corpuscle. × 550; HE TS. Biopsy of a floppy child. Pacinian corpuscles are only rarely seen in muscle biopsies. (d) Pacinian corpuscle. Silver impregnation; teased preparation × 140. The central part of the receptor contains the sensory nerve fibre, sensitive to pressure deformation.

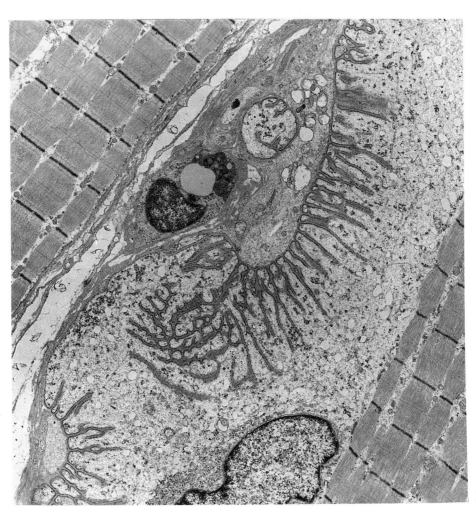

(a)

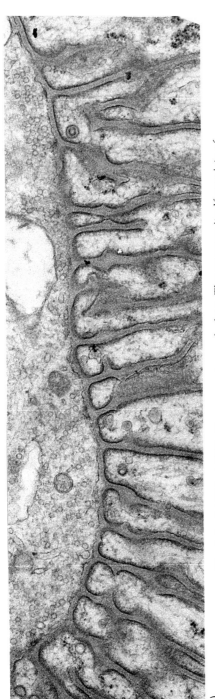

Fig. 3.6 (a) EM × 9860. Human motor end-plate. The synapse itself consists of primary and secondary postsynaptic clefts lined by basement membrane, situated on an axonal hillock of mitochondria-rich cytoplasm. The terminal axonal swelling is seen as it approaches the end-plate zone.
(b) EM × 44 000. The acetylcholinergic vesicles of the presynaptic portion of the end-plate are clearly seen. M muscle. A axon.

(b)

in association with blood vessels, forming the *neurovascular bundles*. Smaller branches can rarely be recognized without silver impregnations. The nerve bundles contain myelinated fibres of various diameters, including motor axons innervating extrafusal and intrafusal muscle fibres, the alpha and gamma motor fibres, respectively, and large sensory axons innervating sensory receptors in muscle spindles, Golgi tendon organs and Pacinian capsules. Small C fibres mediating pain are also present.

3.4.6   Blood vessels

In the neurovascular bundles small arteries and veins may be found. Within individual fascicles smaller vessels, consisting of arterioles, venules and perimysial capillaries, can be identified. Each muscle fibre is surrounded by 2 to 5 capillaries (Andersson and Henriksson, 1977).

3.4.7   Motor end-plates

Each muscle fibre is in contact with a single motor end-plate. The neuromuscular junction consists of a neural component and a muscular component, but this detail can only be clearly seen with the electron microscope (Fig. 3.6). With the light microscope the soleplate or muscular part of the end-plate consists of a slight elevation of the surface of the muscle fibre often associated with a few 'soleplate nuclei' to form the Doyère eminence. The neural part of the end-plate is separated from the muscle fibre by the synaptic cleft, and consists of short axonal expansions, covered by Schwann cell cytoplasm. This cleft consists of complex, closely apposed synaptic folds in which acetylcholinesterase can be demonstrated. The axonal expansions contain mitochondria and multiple clear synaptic vesicles. Differences between motor end-plates innervating Type 1 and Type 2 muscle fibres have been described (Duchen, 1971) but these cannot readily be recognized without quantitative ultrastructural studies.

Most muscle biopsies do not contain motor end-plates, since it is not common for muscle biopsies to be routinely taken from the region of the end-plate zone, i.e., at the motor point of the muscle. The supravital methylene blue method has been much used to demonstrate the terminal axonal pattern, and the structure of the neural part of the motor end-plates, the subneural apparatus, in research studies of neuromuscular disorders, especially in myasthenia gravis (Coërs and Woolf, 1959). The cholinesterase/silver method is more convenient and is applicable to routine diagnostic work (see Fig. 2.7).

References

Andersson, P. and Henriksson, J. (1977) Capillary supply of the quadriceps femoris muscle of man: Adaptive response to exercise. *J. Physiol. (Lond.)*, **270**, 677–690.

Bell, C.D. and Conen, P.E. (1968) Histopathological changes in Duchenne muscular dystrophy. *J. Neurol. Sci.*, **7**, 529–544.

Blomstrand, E. and Ekblom, B. (1982) The needle biopsy technique for fibre type determination in human skeletal muscle – a methodological study. *Acta Physiol. Scand.*, **116**, 437–442.

Blomstrand, E., Celsing, F., Friden, J. and Eklan, B. (1984) How to calculate human muscle fibre areas in biopsy samples – methodological considerations. *Acta Physiol. Scand.*, **122**, 545–551.

Brooke, M.H. and Engel, W.K. (1969) The histographic analysis of human muscle biopsies with regard to fiber types. 1. Adult male and female. *Neurology*, **19**, 221–233.

Coërs, C. and Woolf, A.L. (1959) *The Innervation of Muscle: a Biopsy Study*, Blackwell Scientific Publications, Oxford.

Dubowitz, V. (1985) *Muscle Biopsy – a practical approach*. Bailliere Tindall, London.

Duchen, L.W. (1971) An electron microscope comparison of motor end-plates of slow and fast skeletal muscle fibres of the mouse. *J. Neurol. Sci.*, **14**, 37–45.

Edgerton, V.R. (1970) Morphology and histochemistry of the soleus muscle from normal and exercised rats. *Am. J. Anat.*, **127**, 81–87.

Edstrom, L. and Grimby, L. (1986) Effects of exercise on the motor unit. *Muscle Nerve*, **9**, 104–126.

Edstrom, L. and Kugelberg, E. (1968) Histochemical composition, distribution of fibres and fatiguability of single motor units. *J. Neurol. Neurosurg. Psychiatry*, **31**, 424–433.

Greenfield, J.G., Shy, G.M., Alvord, E.C. and Berg, L. (1957) *An Atlas of Muscle Pathology in Neuromuscular Diseases*, Churchill Livingstone, Edinburgh.

Hall-Craggs, E.C.B. (1970) The longitudinal division of fibres in over-loaded rat skeletal muscle. *J. Anat.*, **107**, 459–470.

Komi, P.V., Viitasalo, J.H.T., Havu, M. *et al.* (1977) Skeletal muscle fibres and muscle enzyme activities in monozygous and dizygous twins of both sexes. *Acta Physiol. Scand.*, **100**, 385–392.

Lexell, J. and Taylor, C.S. (1989) Variability in muscle fibre areas in whole human quadriceps muscle. How much and why? *Acta Physiol. Scand.*, **136**, 561–568.

Mahon, M., Toman, A., Willan, P.L.T. and Bagnall, K.M. (1984) Variability of histochemical and morphometric data from needle biopsy specimens of human quadriceps femoris muscle. *J. Neurol. Sci.*, **63**, 85–100.

Polgar, J., Johnson, M.A., Weightman, D. and Appleton, D. (1973) Data on fibre size in thirty-six human muscles: an autopsy study. *J. Neurol. Sci.*, **19**, 307–318.

Rubinstein, L.F. (1960) Ageing changes in muscle. In *Structure and Function of Muscle*, Vol. 3 (ed. G.H. Bourne), Academic Press, London, ch. 7, pp. 209–226.

Salmons, S. and Henriksson, J. (1981) The adaptive response of skeletal muscle to increased use. *Muscle Nerve*, **4**, 94–105.

Saltin, B., Nazar, K., Costill, D.C. *et al.* (1976) The nature of the training response: peripheral and central adaptations to one-legged exercise. *Acta Physiol. Scand.*, **96**, 289–305.

Slavin, G., Sowter, C., Ward, P. and Paton, K. (1982) Measurement of striated muscle fibre diameters using interactive computer-aided microscopy. *J. Clin. Pathol.*, **35**, 1268–1271.

Stanstedt, P., Nordell, L.-E. and Henriksson, K.-G. (1982) Quantitative analysis of muscle biopsies from volunteers and patients with neuromuscular disorders. *Acta Neurol. Scand.*, **66**, 130–144.

Swash, M. (1990) Muscle spindle pathology. In *Skeletal Muscle Pathology* (eds F. Mastaglia and J.N. Walton), 2nd edn, Churchill Livingstone, Edinburgh.

Swash, M. and Fox, K.P. (1972a) The effect of age on human skeletal muscle: studies of the morphology and innervation of muscle spindles. *J. Neurol. Sci.*, **16**, 417–432.

Swash, M. and Fox, K.P. (1972b) Techniques for the demonstration of human muscle spindle innervation in neuromuscular disease. *J. Neurol. Sci.*, **15**, 291–302.

Willison, R.G. (1980) Arrangement of muscle fibers of a single motor unit in mammalian muscle. *Muscle Nerve*, **3**, 360–361.

4 Histological features of myopathic and neurogenic disorders

It is usually not difficult to decide whether a muscle biopsy is normal or abnormal. Minor abnormalities such as slight changes in fibre size, or a slight increase in central nucleation, which may only be recognized by morphometric and statistical analysis, are not generally important in diagnosis, unless they are accompanied by other, more obvious changes. However, in some conditions such as McArdle's disease and myo-adenylate deaminase deficiency the routine histological and enzyme histochemical techniques may not reveal any striking abnormality, the diagnosis being recognized only when special techniques are applied. Occasionally a muscle biopsy may be normal because an uninvolved muscle has inadvertently been selected for biopsy. It is not appropriate, or economic, to try to investigate every biopsy with a complete range of histochemical techniques. A decision as to how far to pursue the investigation must be made on the basis of clinical information and the results of laboratory tests, in addition to the findings on the routine histological and enzyme histological methods. Histological abnormalities almost invariably accompany weakness.

The clinical findings and the results of laboratory and electro-physiological tests usually indicate whether the patient's muscular symptoms, especially weakness, are due to myopathic or neurogenic disease, but difficulties often arise in the investigation of patients with proximal muscular weakness. In these patients the distinction can only be made by muscle biopsy (Black *et al.*, 1974). The abnormalities found in myopathic and neurogenic disorders overlap to some extent, and this can lead to difficulties if enzyme histochemical techniques are not used. The recognition of the frequency of spinal muscular atrophy in patients presenting with proximal weakness stems from use of these methods. Formerly, most of these patients were considered to be suffering from limb-girdle muscular dystrophy. Despite these areas of overlap there are certain cardinal features of myopathic and neurogenic disorders and these are of great importance in diagnosis.

The first step in diagnosis, having recognized that a muscle biopsy is abnormal, is to decide whether the abnormality is *myopathic* or *neurogenic*; this decision can only be made with certainty after study of the enzyme histochemical techniques, particularly the NADH and ATPase preparations.

4.1 Myopathic disorders

The main histological features of myopathic disorders are shown in Table 4.1. The general features shown in this table are abnormalities characteristic of myopathies, especially in inherited muscular dystrophies and inflammatory or toxic myopathies. In metabolic myopathies, on the other hand, fibre necrosis and regeneration are relatively uncommon, although other features, especially Type 2 fibre atrophy, central nucleation and increased variability in fibre size, may be present. Many myopathies, especially the myopathies of childhood, are recognized by the occurrence of specific morphological changes within muscle fibres, and these may be virtually the only abnormality in the biopsy. These specific abnormalities will be discussed in later chapters.

4.1.1   Muscle fibre necrosis

Necrosis is a common and fundamental feature of many myopathies. It may result from a variety of factors, including trauma, heat, cold, vascular

Table 4.1   Histological features of myopathies

General features
   Single fibre necrosis, and regeneration
   Increased variability in fibre size, including hypertrophy and/or atrophy
   Increased central nucleation
   Selective Type 2 fibre atrophy
   Type 1 fibre predominance
   Fibre splitting
   Endomysial fibrosis and fat replacement of muscle fibres
   Changes in myofibrillar pattern, e.g. whorled fibres and moth-eaten fibres
   Fibre-type grouping uncommon

Features specific to certain myopathies
   Perivascular and endomysial mononuclear cell infiltration
   Perifascicular atrophy
   Various specific morphological abnormalities in muscle fibres, e.g. hyaline fibres, rod bodies, ragged-red fibres, central cores, tubular aggregates
   Abnormalities in blood vessels
   Muscle spindle abnormalities, e.g. myotonic dystrophy

insufficiency, drugs and toxins, and all these factors have been used experimentally to study the initial histological features of necrosis and the sequence of regenerative changes that follow. The well-known descriptions of muscle fibre necrosis, consisting of vacuolation, hyaline changes, and Zenker's waxy degeneration (Zenker, 1864), are based on the appearances seen in paraffin-embedded material. In frozen sections the histological features differ somewhat from this pattern, largely because of the absence of fixation-induced changes.

A sequence of changes occurs in necrotic fibres (Figs 4.1 and 4.2). The earliest abnormality recognizable by light microscopy is a loss of granularity, producing an amorphous eosinophilic appearance in HE preparations (Fig. 4.1). At this stage the ATPase reactivity is unchanged, since myofibrils remain *in situ*, but with SDH or NADH the fibre appears either less reactive than normal, due to loss of mitochondrial enzymes, or appears floccular. Later, areas of patchy pallor can be seen in HE preparations. This is accompanied by pallor of nuclei and by the appearance of DNA in the sarcoplasm; acid phosphatase and RNA can

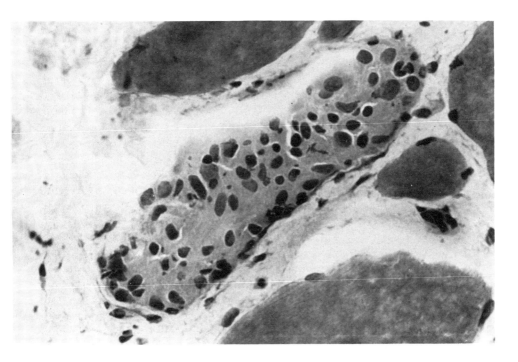

Fig. 4.1 × 427; HE. Necrosis of this fibre has proceeded to macrophage infiltration. The ultrastructural counterpart of this phase of fibre necrosis is shown in Fig. 4.6.

usually also be demonstrated at this time. Infiltration by macrophages follows, usually leaving the basement membrane intact. Regeneration (see below) then begins.

Segmental necrosis is a term used to refer to necrosis of only part of a fibre. This can sometimes be recognized in single transverse sections, but is more usually seen in longitudinal sections. When necrosis results from vascular factors, or from 'toxic' effects, as in some drug-induced myopathies, e.g. that due to epsilon aminocaproic acid (Swash and Schwartz, 1983), widespread simultaneous necrosis of many muscle

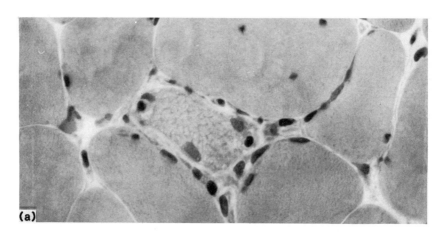

(a)

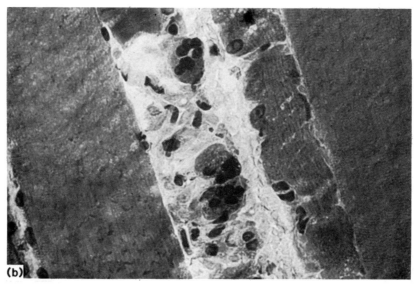

(b)

fibres may occur (Fig. 4.3). The basement membrane and endomysium is usually unaffected in this form of necrosis, so that empty, or macrophage-filled, endomysial tubes remain (subendomysial necrosis).

In other myopathies, especially muscular dystrophies, and poly-myositis, necrotic fibres are found scattered through the biopsy or in clusters in different part of the biopsy. Infiltration of necrotic fibres by macrophages requires adequate capillary perfusion. In some cases of inflammatory myopathies this does not occur and in this situation necrotic muscle fibres may remain more or less intact, but show marked loss of enzyme activity. These are sometimes called *ghost fibres* (Fig. 4.4).

Hyaline fibres have been considered as a special type of muscle fibre necrosis. This abnormality, which is a particularly prominent feature of Duchenne muscular dystrophy (Fig. 4.5), is due to localized hyper-contraction induced by an influx of intracellular calcium entering the

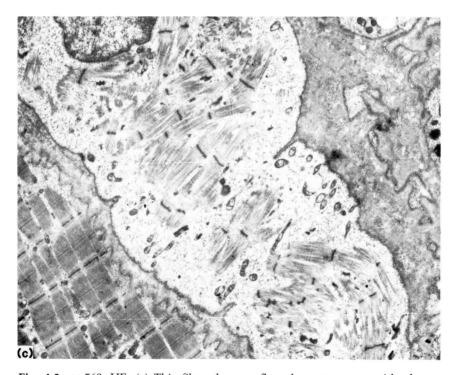

Fig. 4.2 × 560; HE. (a) This fibre shows a floccular appearance with plump nuclei. This probably represents regeneration following necrosis. (b) In this longitudinal section the necrotic fibre also contains several early regenerating myoblasts. (c) × 6000; EM. Necrotic fibre adjacent to normal fibre. The disarrayed myofibrils and mitochondria may represent an early stage of regeneration.

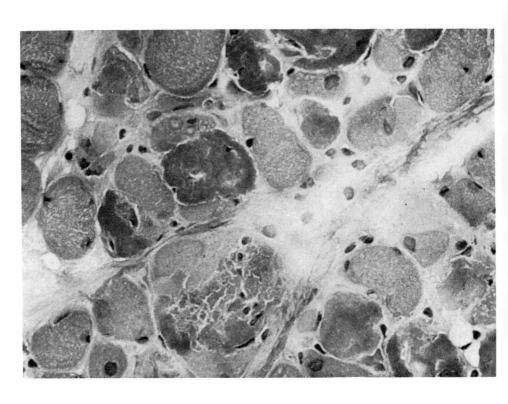

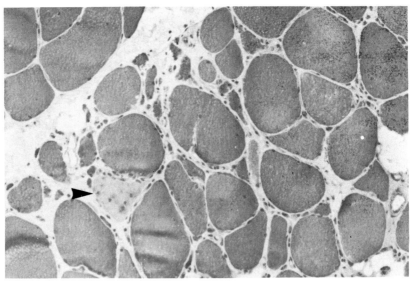

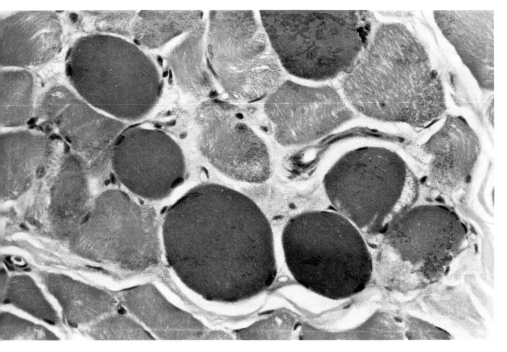

Fig. 4.5 × 405; HE. Duchenne muscular dystrophy. The large, rounded intensely eosinophilic fibres in this paraffin-embedded section have undergone hyaline change.

fibre through defects in the plasma membrane. This excess intracellular calcium induces calcium-dependent proteases leading to death of the cell.

Ultrastructural studies of muscle fibre necrosis have revealed that mitochondrial changes are marked in the early stages. The myofilaments degenerate later, forming amorphous masses of electron-dense material, and the sarcotubular system becomes disorganized. During macrophage

Fig. 4.3 Acute myopathy due to epsilon aminocaproic acid. × 380; HE. Widespread floccular necrosis of muscle fibres, with continuous regeneration occurring from subendomysial crescents, probably representing a satellite cell origin for the regeneration (see Kennard *et al.* (1980)).

Fig. 4.4 × 350; HE. Chronic polymyositis. The 'ghost' fibre (arrow) is pale and amorphous, and contains pale nuclei, probably those of macrophages; these are features of necrosis.

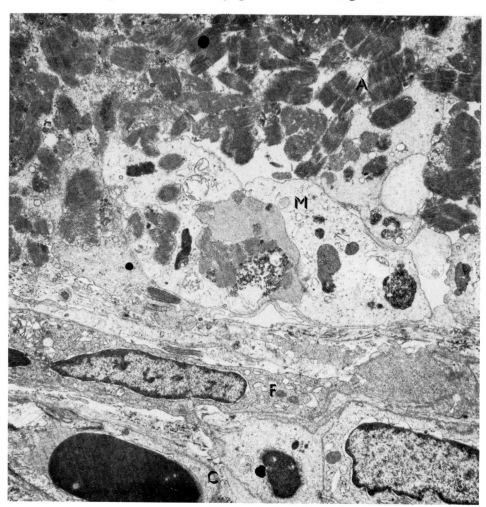

Fig. 4.6   EM × 8750. Polymyositis. The necrotic fibre contains a macrophage (M) within its sarcoplasm. This cell contains electron-dense lysosomal inclusions, and it lacks a basement membrane. The myofilaments are broken up into A band segments (A), and Z and I band material is absent. Outside the fibre, fibroblast cell processes (F) and capillaries (C) are seen.

ingestion the myofilaments tend to become broken into small pieces, consisting of A band material; Z and I band material cannot be identified (Fig. 4.6). This is a feature of necrosis following damage to the fibre's plasma membrane (Cullen and Fulthorpe, 1982). Initially myofilamentous breakdown and loss may be focal within a fibre.

4.1.2   *Muscle fibre regeneration*

Regeneration occurs after necrosis or injury in most tissues of the body and muscle fibres, which are particularly susceptible to injury in everyday life, have considerable regenerative potential. In muscle biopsies it is common to find both necrotic and regenerating fibres in close proximity, indicating that degeneration and repair are occurring concurrently.

Regenerative changes. After fibre necrosis, regeneration can occur either in continuity with the undamaged portions of the fibre ('continuous' repair) or from myoblast formation in the necrotic segment itself ('discontinuous' repair). Regeneration begins at a stage when phagocytosis of necrotic material is still incomplete. At this time mononucleated cells are still abundant in the interstitium around the necrotic fibre.

In 'continuous' regeneration, surviving muscle nuclei become enlarged and vesicular about 4 days after injury, and migrate to the centre of the fibre. The surrounding cytoplasm becomes basophilic, losing its striations and by the 5th–10th day after injury ribbons of basophilic, foamy non-striated sarcoplasm can be seen in the necrotic segment. In 'discontinuous' regeneration, regeneration proceeds from mononucleated myoblasts. These form a component of the basophilic fusiform cells found along the inner surface of the basement membrane of necrotic muscle fibres. Several days after injury these cells form long basophilic multinucleated ribbons which later fuse, forming a new fibre. These ribbons of differentiating sarcoplasm are similar to the myotubes formed during embryonic myogenesis.

The origin of myoblasts during regeneration is controversial (Fig. 4.7). They could arise by segregation from the damaged myofibre itself, by activation of satellite cells pre-existing in the sarcolemmal sheath, or by metaplasia from circulating mesenchymal cells. The weight of evidence (Resnik, 1973) favours the first and second of these suggestions. In particular, the role of satellite cells in regeneration after injury has received support from the observation of activation of these cells after a variety of experimental and naturally occurring modes of fibre injury. Satellite cells are found in normal muscle fibres as a nucleus, surrounded by sparse granular sarcoplasm containing abundant free ribosomes, Golgi apparatus, endoplasmic reticulum and mitochondria, but devoid of any myofilaments. The satellite cell is limited by plasma membrane, and is situated beneath the basement membrane of the muscle fibre. The numbers of such cells in muscle are increased after injury (Resnik, 1973) and after denervation (Ontell, 1974). Resnik (1973) has reviewed the ultrastructural sequence of changes giving rise to myoblast formation in these cells during regeneration after cold-induced injury.

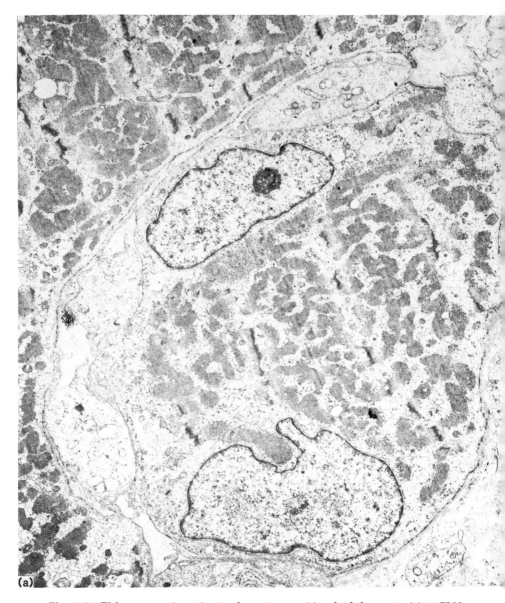

Fig. 4.7 EM regeneration. Acute dermatomyositis of adult onset. (a) × 7200. Regeneration from satellite cells results in myoblast formations so that several maturing muscle fibres appear enclosed by a single sarcolemmal tube (basal lamina) although each has its own plasma membrane tube. The nuclei show a dispersed chromatin pattern and the myofibrils are contained in a granular sarcoplasm. Variations in maturity of myofibrillar development are apparent.

Webb (1977) has drawn attention to the importance of programmed cell death of myotubes during embryonic myogenesis. The stimulus for cell death is probably muscle cell activity, and a similar phenomenon probably occurs during differentiation of myoblasts in regenerative repair, since large numbers of developing myotubes are found in the early stages of repair, before fusion occurs and the single myofibre is reconstituted. The achievement of functional reinnervation, which can only occur when the fibre is reconstituted across the necrotic segment, is important in this process (Fig. 4.8).

In muscle biopsies regenerating fibres have a characteristic appearance (Fig. 4.8). The sarcoplasm appears basophilic and granular, and it often contains copious small lipid droplets. The sarcoplasmic nuclei are usually large and vesicular with prominent nucleoli and a dispersed chromatin pattern. The myofibrillar density is low so that myofibrillar enzymes, such as the myofibrillar ATPase, may be poorly reactive. These fibres often express the enzymatic features of Type 2C fibres (see Table 2.4). The basophilic sarcoplasm of regenerating fibres shows increased RNA content, and increased acid phosphatase activity (Neerunjun and Dubowitz, 1977). Regenerating fibres express fetal myosin (Sartore *et al.*, 1982) and contain increased amounts of desmin protein (Thornell *et al.*, 1980). Sometimes these changes are seen in only part of the transverse diameter of a fibre. Regenerating fibres often occur in small groups and, even if single, they are usually smaller than normal fibres.

4.1.3   Increased variability in fibre size

In normal muscle most muscle fibres are 40–80 μm in diameter in men, and 30–70 μm in diameter in women (see Chapter 3). It is characteristic of myopathic disorders that many fibres, larger or smaller than the normal range, occur in the biopsy and in some disorders; for example, in limb-girdle muscular dystrophy, very large (>120 μm) and very small (<20 μm) fibres may occur. Histograms of fibre diameter in such biopsies demonstrate the wide range of diameters. This increased variability in fibre size is due to hypertrophy, probably occurring as a compensatory response to the increased load imposed on surviving healthy muscle fibres in muscles in which loss of functioning muscle fibres has occurred (Swash and Schwartz, 1977), and to atrophy. Atrophy results from incomplete regeneration, from necrosis, or from fibre splitting. Increased variability in fibre size may be the most striking abnormality in relatively mild non-progressive myopathies; this often reflects selective atrophy of a fibre type, usually of Type 2 fibres as in many metabolic myopathies.

4.1.4   Increased central nucleation

Central nucleation is common in myopathies (Fig. 4.9). It usually occurs in hypertrophied fibres but it is also found in small basophilic regenerating fibres (Fig. 4.10). In hypertrophied fibres multiple central nuclei are often seen, and these are sometimes associated with clefts or splits in the sarcoplasm of the fibre. Multiple central nucleation in fibres of normal size is a feature of myotonic dystrophy. In normal muscle up to 3% of the fibres may contain central nuclei.

4.1.5   Selective Type 2 fibre atrophy

In myopathies selective atrophy of Type 2 fibres is a common finding (Fig. 4.11). However, this is not a specific feature of myopathies since it is found also in disuse atrophy, in patients with stroke and in Parkinson's disease. Occasionally, especially in steroid myopathy, Type 2 atrophy may be so marked that the atrophic fibres appear thin and pointed, resembling acute denervation. Unless ATPase preparations are made this selective involvement cannot be recognized. In most myopathies the Type 2B fibres are more atrophic than the Type 2A fibres.

4.1.6   Type 1 fibre predominance

Fibre-type predominance is not in itself a specific abnormality, and the selection implied in small needle biopsies may make it difficult to assess. However, Type 1 fibre predominance (> 55% Type 1 fibres) is, in general, associated with myopathies, particularly Duchenne dystrophy and childhood myopathies. It is also found in about a third of biopsies from patients with limb-girdle muscular dystrophy.

When a biopsy contains a large proportion of fibres of one histochemical type caution must be exercised in assessing whether or not there is fibre-type grouping, since fibres of a single type will inevitably be found in proximity to each other (Johnson *et al.*, 1973). Fibre-type grouping can only be recognized with certainty when groups of both Type 1 and Type 2 fibres occur.

Fig. 4.8   Regeneration (a) × 380; HE. Regenerating subendomysial myoblasts have differentiated but have not yet fused to form single new fibres. The perimysium separates a regenerating fascicle from an adjacent nearly normal fascicle in this patient with acute polymyositis. (b) × 380; ATPase, pH 4.3. Serial section to (a). The regenerating subendomysial fibre clusters are clearly seen. Some fibres are of intermediate type (Type 2C).

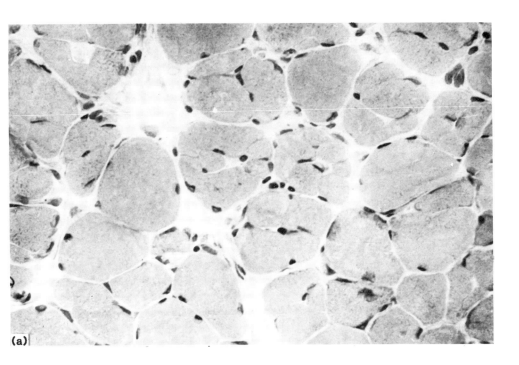

(a)

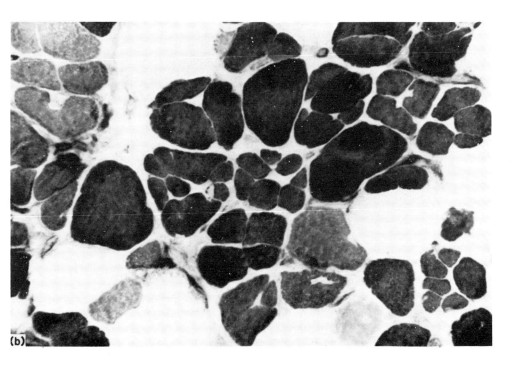

(b)

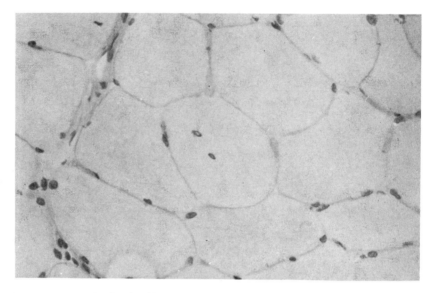

Fig. 4.9 × 350; PAS. The fibre in the middle of the field contains two centrally-placed nuclei, and another fibre contains a single centrally-placed nucleus.

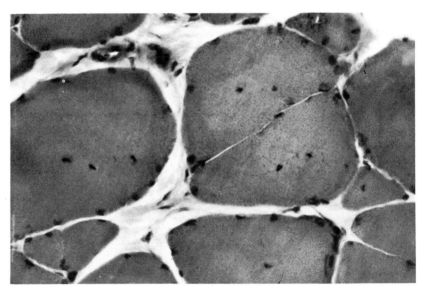

Fig. 4.10 × 350; HE. Polymyositis. These hypertrophied fibres, greater than 100 μm diameter, contain multiple central nuclei. There is a moderate increase in the amount of endomysial fibrous tissue.

4.1.7 Fibre splitting

Hypertrophied fibres are particularly likely to show fibre splitting (Fig. 4.12). The split usually begins at the periphery of the fibre and is directed toward a centrally located nucleus, but in some instances the split may consist solely of a central cleft associated with nearby nuclei. The cleft at the edges of the frank zone of splitting is usually basophilic and the nuclei associated with this cleft appear vesicular. The longitudinal extent of splits varies but extends up to about 150 μm (Schwartz *et al.*, 1976). Some clefts contain a capillary (Sulaiman and Kinder, 1989) and these tend to be longer, extending up to 1200 μm, and to be found in distal leg muscles. Sometimes a fibre may be split into multiple fragments. Fibre splitting is a normal phenomenon near musculotendinous insertions and it must not be confused with subendomysial regeneration which occurs in association with fibre necrosis. Muscle fibre splitting is a common feature of muscular dystrophies and it is also found in chronic polymyositis. It is also a feature of long-standing neurogenic disorders in which secondary myopathic changes have developed (Schwartz *et al.*, 1976). *Ring fibres* can be interpreted as a special example of splitting in which one or more myofibrils become displaced from their normal longitudinal orientation to take up a spirally arranged location around the main group of myofibrils (Fig. 4.13).

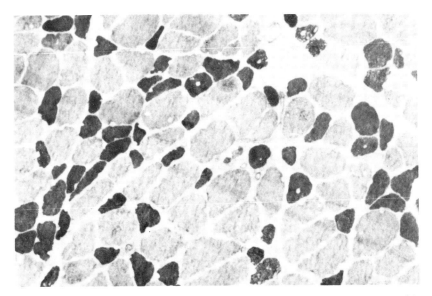

Fig. 4.11 $\times$ 140; ATPase. Steroid myopathy. The dark Type 2 fibres are atrophic; and the pale Type 1 fibres are of normal size.

4.1.8   *Endomysial fibrosis and fatty replacement*

These features represent a feature of the advanced stages of myopathic disease. Marked fibrosis is especially prominent in Duchenne muscular dystrophy, and fatty replacement of muscular tissue represents the late stages of disease, when compensatory processes have failed and regenerative repair no longer occurs.

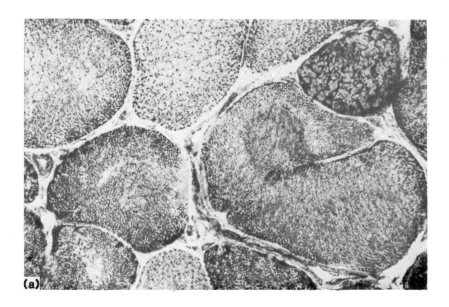

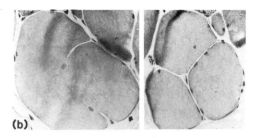

Fig. 4.12   Fibre splitting. (a) × 560; NADH. A cleft of splitting invaginates the large fibre and almost bisects it. This process is often associated with a centrally located nucleus. (b) × 120; HE. Serial sections 80 μm apart to show the relation of fibre splitting to central nuclei. (c) EM × 14 250. Longitudinal section. A cleft lined by plasma membrane and basement membrane invaginates the fibre, directed downward toward the nucleus.

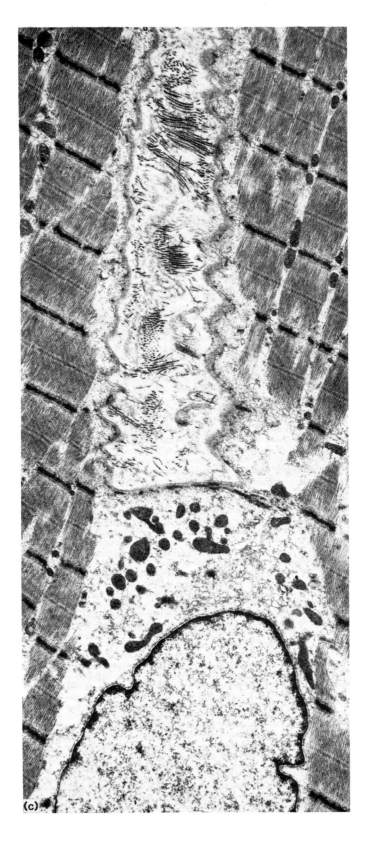

(c)

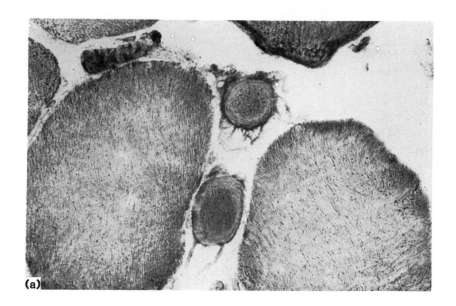

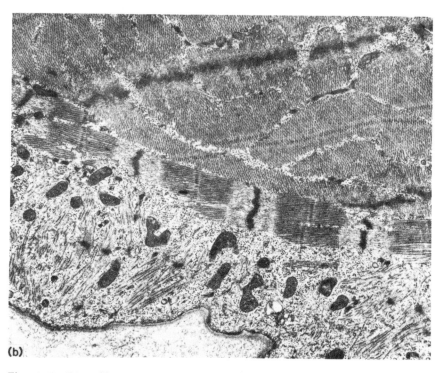

Fig. 4.13 Ring fibres (a) × 560; NADH. Two small fibres show displaced peripherally located myofibrils. This is a non-specific abnormality. (b) × 15 000; EM. Myotonic dystrophy. A ring-like displaced myofibril encircles the fibre.

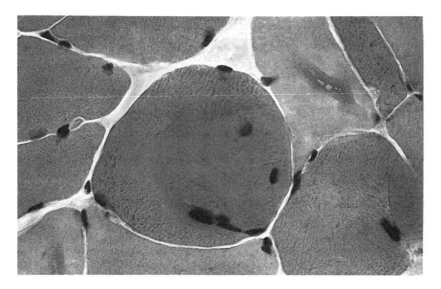

Fig. 4.14 Whorled fibre – HE. × 500. There is whorled pattern in the sarcoplasm of the fibre. This is a non-specific abnormality.

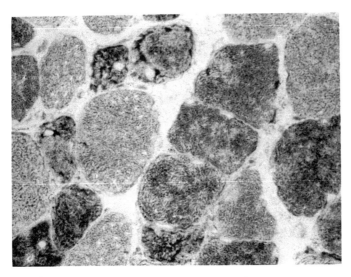

Fig. 4.15 Polymyositis. Lobulated and moth-eaten fibres. × 380. NADH. There are zones of poor enzyme reactivity and the Type 1 fibres have a lobulated appearance.

4.1.9   Whorled, moth-eaten fibres and lobulated fibres

Changes in myofibrillar organization occur especially in limb-girdle muscular dystrophy syndromes and in inflammatory myopathies. In NADH preparations these abnormalities are demonstrated by the distortion of the normal speckled pattern of mitochondrial reactivity (Figs 4.14 and 4.15).

4.1.10   Features specific to certain myopathies

These are described in relation to the disorder in which they are the predominant feature.

4.2   Neurogenic disorders

The main histological features of neurogenic disorders are shown in Table 4.2. In neurogenic disorders the histological features are not specific for particular disorders, since the changes in the muscle are themselves due to loss of innervation (*denervation*) or to *reinnervation* after denervation. Neurogenic disorders may be acute or chronic and many of the latter may continue for many years; for example the familial neuropathies and spinal muscular atrophies. In these long-standing neurogenic disorders secondary myopathic changes may develop in affected muscles, in addition to neurogenic changes.

4.2.1   Histological features of denervation

After denervation muscle fibres undergo atrophy. This atrophy is a slow process reaching its peak in about 4 months after interruption to the nerve supply. In most neurogenic disorders, however, denervation is neither total nor of abrupt onset. Rather, the disease is progressive and of gradual onset, so that muscle fibres belonging to one motor unit in a muscle may

Table 4.2   Histological features of neurogenic disorders

Denervation
    Disseminated neurogenic atrophy
    Target fibres
    Grouped neurogenic atrophy
    Changes in intramuscular nerve bundles

Reinnervation
    Fibre-type grouping
    Fibre-type predominance

be denervated while muscle fibres forming part of an adjacent motor unit may still have a normal innervation. There is thus a wide variation in the state of innervation, and in the stage of the neurogenic process in individual muscles. The histological appearances in neurogenic disorders reflect these processes.

After nerve section the first change in a muscle is increased roundness of the sarcolemmal nuclei, which develop prominent nucleoli. After about 2 weeks an increase in central nucleation is evident. Reduction in muscle fibre diameter becomes detectable after about 4 weeks and after 2 months the muscle fibre diameter is reduced to about half normal. The striations, however, are still present. Atrophy reaches its peak between the third and fourth months after denervation, and these muscle fibres tend to assume a polygonal or pointed shape at about this stage, or later. At this stage, i.e. more than 6 months after denervation, the muscle fibres are small (< 20 μm diameter) and the sarcolemmal nuclei are small, dark and pyknotic (Adams *et al.*, 1953). Even after nerve section, however, some muscle fibres are relatively more resistant to denervation atrophy than others. Target fibres are a special feature of acute denervation (see below).

(a) *Disseminated neurogenic atrophy*. The minimal detectable abnormality in a neurogenic disorder, using histological techniques, consists of single

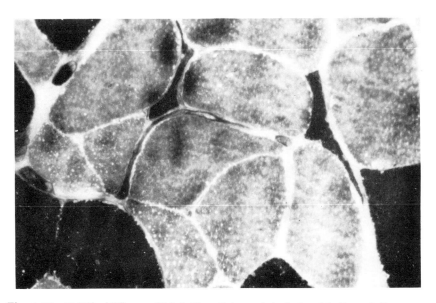

Fig. 4.16 × 560; ATPase, pH 9.4. Two thin, pointed atrophic Type 2 fibres are surrounded by normal Type 1 and Type 2 fibres; *disseminated neurogenic atrophy*.

atrophic muscle fibres, or small clusters of atrophic fibres, found scattered through the biopsy (Fig. 4.16). These atrophic fibres appear thin and pointed, and react strongly in NADH preparations so that they appear abnormally dark with this technique (Fig. 4.17). They also react positively in non-specific esterase preparations. With myofibrillar ATPase they may be of either major histochemical type. They usually contain dark, pyknotic nuclei and these may be multiple in a single cross-section. They do not show marked acid phosphatase activity and they are not basophilic.

These atrophic fibres represent muscle fibres denervated by damage to a single motor axon or to its terminal twigs. They are therefore found in muscle biopsies both in anterior horn cell diseases, and in motor neuropathies.

(b) *Grouped neurogenic atrophy*. This consists of groups of small atrophic fibres, of the same histochemical type in myofibrillar ATPase preparations (Fig. 4.18). The fibres in each group are generally of similar size and may represent part or the whole of a fascicle. The individual atrophic fibres in grouped neurogenic atrophy (Fig. 4.18) show the same histological and histochemical features, particularly the prominent reactivity in SDH and NADH preparations, as do the atrophic fibres in

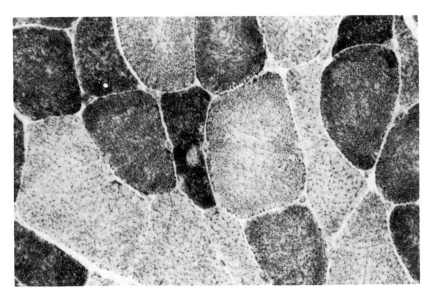

Fig. 4.17   × 560; NADH. The central narrow, darkly-reactive fibre contains a target zone consisting of a pale central area rimmed with positively reacting material; *target fibre* abnormality.

disseminated neurogenic atrophy; they thus show the histological features of denervation. The significance of grouped denervation atrophy is that it implies that denervation has occurred after reinnervation (see *Fibre-type grouping* below) and it is therefore a phenomenon representing a relatively decompensated, and later stage, of a progressive neurogenic disorder.

(c) *Target fibres*. These consist of fibres containing abnormalities in their centres best seen in myofibrillar ATPase and NADH preparations (Fig. 4.19). The abnormality consists of a central, unstained zone surrounded by a densely stained intermediate zone and a third relatively normal outer zone extending to the edge of the fibre. Type 1 fibres are preferentially affected. Target fibres are found in acutely denervated muscle, especially in peripheral nerve lesions, such as nerve transections and acute neuropathies, but they may sometimes be found in rapidly progressive anterior horn cell disease, e.g. motor neuron disease. Although a characteristic feature of denervation they can be produced experimentally by tenotomy (Engel *et al.*, 1966).

(d) *Changes in intramuscular nerve bundles*. Biopsies often contain intramuscular nerve bundles and, in the presence of marked neurogenic change, these nerve fascicles may themselves show abnormalities of diagnostic value. For example, Wallerian degeneration and Schwann cell hyperplasia can easily be recognized in axonal neuropathies and certain demyelinating neuropathies, respectively.

4.2.2 *Histological features of reinnervation*

Reinnervation after denervation may occur, in favourable circumstances, e.g. in acute neuropathies, by regeneration of axons to reinnervate the motor end-plates of the denervated fibres before severe and irreversible muscle fibre atrophy has occurred.

In most progressive neurogenic disorders, however, muscle fibre reinnervation occurs by collateral axonal sprouting from nearby axons representing the terminal neuronal tree of a different anterior horn cell from that originally innervating these muscle fibres (Wohlfart, 1957; 1958). Because of the intermingling of muscle fibres belonging to different motor units in the muscle, such collateral sprouts may be only a few hundred micrometres long. Further, collateral reinnervation may result in a muscle fibre receiving new innervation from a motor unit of different histochemical type, thus inducing this muscle fibre to change its histochemical type and resulting in enlargement of the residual motor units. As more fibres become reinnervated by this process, small groups of reinnervated fibres of the same histological type can be identified in the biopsy. Each reinnervated fibre receives innervation from a single axon, as in normal muscle.

Several factors prejudice the development of effective reinnervation. These include prominent muscle fibre atrophy prior to the arrival of collateral sprouts in the vicinity of the denervated fibres and failure of denervated fibres to receive collateral axonal sprouts either because of deficient capacity to sprout, due to metabolic abnormalities in neuronal or axonal cytoplasm, or because of physical factors in the muscle itself such as fibrous tissue barriers. Wohlfart (1957) estimated that collateral axonal sprouting is so effective that as many as 30% of anterior horn cells can be lost in motor neuron disease before weakness becomes clinically apparent. In such a muscle there would be marked histological evidence of reinnervation.

(a) *Fibre-type grouping*. In normal muscle the muscle fibres belonging to individual motor units are widely distributed within a limited area, up to 20%, of the cross-sectional area of a muscle, so that the fibres of individual motor units intermingle and their territories overlap (Edstrom and Kugelberg, 1968). Fibres belonging to a single motor unit are thus usually isolated but sometimes two or four such fibres are adjacent to each other, and occasionally up to six fibres occur together in a straight or curved row (Edstrom and Kugelberg, 1968). When reinnervation occurs by collateral axonal sprouting small or large groups of fibres of the same histochemical

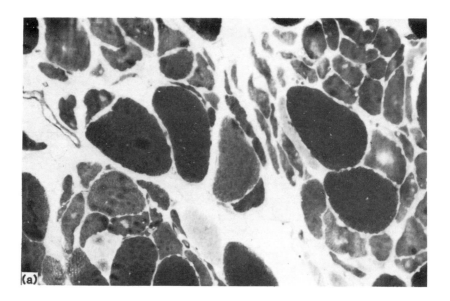

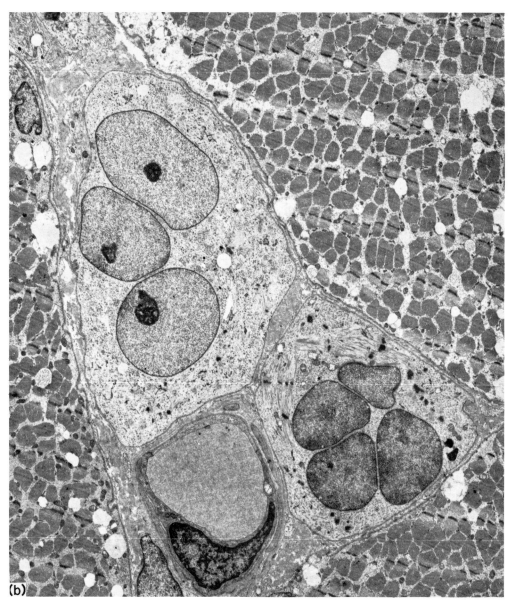

Fig. 4.18 (a) × 350; ATPase pH 9.4. In the centre of the field is a group of narrow atrophic fibres; *small grouped atrophy*. (b) EM × 4200. Two denervated fibres. Note the prominent nuclei and the sparse degenerate myofilamentous material. There is a capillary nearby.

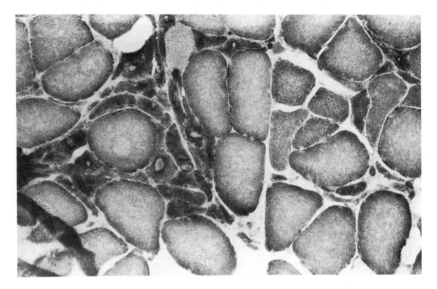

Fig. 4.19   × 350; NADH. A group of atrophic, darkly-reactive fibres (*grouped denervation atrophy*) show target formations.

type are formed; *fibre-type grouping*. In experimental studies fibre-type grouping does not occur earlier than 6 weeks after peripheral nerve injury (Warszanski *et al.*, 1975).

   The recognition of fibre-type grouping depends on somewhat arbitrary criteria. Fibre-type grouping is generally defined as the presence of two or more fibres of identical fibre type completely enclosed, at all points on their circumference, by other fibres of the same histochemical type (Fig. 4.20). Since normal muscle fibres tend to be of approximately equal size, and to assume a six-sided configuration (see Willison, 1980), this definition implies that a group of fibres will contain not less than 10 fibres of the same histochemical type. However, the number of fibres required to produce fibre-type grouping will depend, to some extent, on the size of the fibres, particularly the size of the enclosed fibres themselves. If the latter are small, fewer surrounding fibres may be required to enclose them. It is thus an empirical criterion that a group should consist of at least 12 fibres before it can be regarded as significant. Furthermore, the presence of fibre-type grouping of both histochemical fibre types in the biopsy lends weight to the observation, and multiple areas of fibre-type grouping usually occur in well-established neurogenic disorders. A single zone of fibre-type grouping should be interpreted with caution since this may represent a nearby fascicle with a different proportion of one or other fibre type, and not fibre-type grouping.

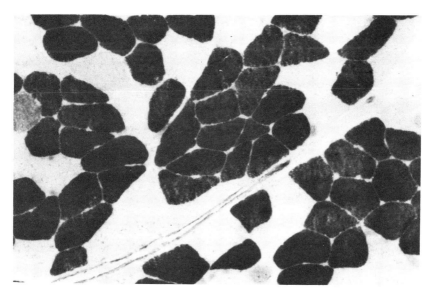

Fig. 4.20 × 140; ATPase, pH 4.3. *Fibre-type grouping.* The central group consists of >12 fibres of the same histochemical type, and three of these fibres are entirely enclosed by fibres of the same type.

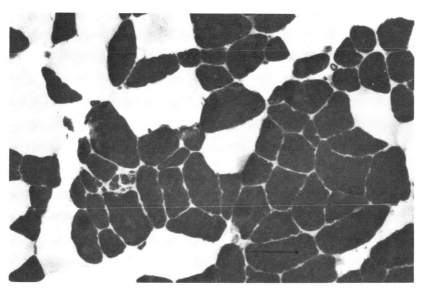

Fig. 4.21 × 140; ATPase, pH 4.3. *Fibre-type predominance.* The majority of the fibres in the field are of the same histochemical type. This appearance may, as in this example, resemble fibre-type grouping. One fibre, undergoing regeneration, appears fragmented.

In muscles in which fibre-type predominance is marked it is difficult to recognize fibre-type grouping, unless the group consists of fibres of the less predominant type. Johnson *et al.* (1973) pointed out that two or more enclosed fibres will commonly occur when a fibre type is predominant by 70% or more.

In fibre-type grouping the fibres within the group usually vary in size, whereas in fibre-type predominance, they tend to be of more nearly uniform size.

(b) *Fibre-type predominance*. Fibre-type predominance may be a feature of neurogenic or myopathic conditions. In neurogenic disorders either fibre type may be predominant, whereas Type 1 fibre predominance is more frequently found in myopathies (Fig. 4.21). In a small biopsy fibre-type predominance may represent a sample of a large group of reinnervated fibres. This is a particular hazard of needle biopsies in which only a small sample of the muscle is available. When fibre-type predominance is found in a muscle such as vastus lateralis or biceps brachii, which normally contain approximately equal numbers of Type 1, Type 2A and Type 2B fibres, it assumes particular significance, and a neurogenic disorder should be suspected.

4.2.3   *Secondary myopathic change in chronic neurogenic disorders*

In long-standing neurogenic disorders such as poliomyelitis, spinal muscular atrophy and hereditary motor neuropathies, histological changes resembling those of myopathies may be found. These myopathic changes pose a difficult problem in diagnosis since they may obscure the underlying neurogenic lesion unless enzyme histochemical techniques are used to demonstrate the presence of denervated fibres, and fibre-type grouping. The most common myopathic features seen in these chronic neurogenic disorders are shown in Table 4.3. These changes occur as part

Table 4.3 'Secondary myopathic' changes in chronic neurogenic disorders (see Cazzato, 1970; Drachman *et al.*, 1967; Haase and Shy, 1960; Schwartz *et al.*, 1976)

Histological evidence of denervation and reinnervation (see Table 4.2) plus:
Increased central nucleation
Longitudinal splitting of muscle fibres
Muscle fibre hypertrophy (mainly Type 1 fibres)
Degenerative changes
Isolated regenerating fibre clusters
Increased variation in fibre size
Interstitial fibrosis

of a sequence of compensatory phenomena in weakened muscles, particularly in relation to fibre hypertrophy and fibre splitting (Schwartz *et al.*, 1976; Swash and Schwartz, 1988).

References

Adams, R.D., Denny-Brown, D. and Pearson, C.M. (1953) *Diseases of Muscle*, Cassell, London.

Black, J.T., Bhatt, G.P., DeJesus, P.V. *et al.* (1974) Diagnostic accuracy of clinical data, quantitative electromyography and histochemistry in neuromuscular disease: a study of 105 cases. *J. Neurol. Sci.*, **21**, 59–70.

Cazzato, G. (1970) Myopathic changes in denervated muscle: a study of biopsy material in various neuromuscular diseases. In *Muscle Diseases* (eds J.N. Walton, N. Canal and G. Scarlato), Exerpta Medica, Amsterdam, pp. 392–401.

Cullen, M.J. and Fulthorpe, J.J. (1982) Phagocytosis of the A band following Z line and I band loss: Its significance in skeletal muscle breakdown. *J. Pathol.*, **138**, 129–143.

Drachman, D.B., Murphy, J.R.N., Nigam, M.P. and Hills, J.R. (1967) 'Myopathic' changes in chronically denervated muscle. *Arch. Neurol.*, **16**, 14–24.

Edstrom, L. and Kugelberg, E. (1968) Histochemical composition, distribution of fibres and fatiguability of single motor units. *J. Neurol. Neurosurg. Psychiatry*, **31**, 424–433.

Engel, W.K., Brooke, M.H. and Nelson, P.G. (1966) Histochemical studies of denervated or tenotomised cat muscle. *Ann. NY Acad. Sci.*, **138**, 160–185.

Haase, G.R. and Shy, G.M. (1960) Pathological changes in muscle biopsies from patients with peroneal muscle atrophy. *Brain*, **83**, 631–637.

Johnson, M.A., Polgar, J., Weightman, D. and Appleton, D. (1973) Data on the distribution of fibre types in thirty six human muscles: an autopsy study. *J. Neurol. Sci.*, **18**, 111–129.

Neerunjun, S.J.S. and Dubowitz, V. (1977) Concomitance of basophilia, ribonucleic acid and acid phosphatase activity in regenerating muscle fibres. *J. Neurol. Sci.*, **33**, 95–109.

Ontell, M. (1974) Muscle satellite cells. *Anat. Rec.*, **178**, 211–228.

Resnik, M. (1973) Current concepts of skeletal muscle regeneration. In *The Striated Muscle* (ed. C.M. Pearson), Williams and Wilkins, Baltimore, pp. 185–225.

Sartore, S., Gorza, L. and Schiaffino, S. (1982) Fetal myosin heavy chains in regenerating muscle. *Nature*, **298**, 294–296.

Schwartz, M.S., Sargeant, M.K. and Swash, M. (1976) Longitudinal fibre splitting in neurogenic muscular disorders – its relation to the pathogenesis of myopathic change. *Brain*, **99**, 617–636.

Sulaiman, A.R. and Kinder, D.S. (1989) Vascularised muscle fibres: etiopathogenesis and clinical significance. *J. Neurol. Sci.*, **92**, 37–54.

Swash, M. and Schwartz, M.S. (1977) Implications of longitudinal muscle fibre splitting in neurogenic and myopathic disorders. *J. Neurol. Neurosurg. Psychiatry*, **40**, 1152–1159.

Swash, M. and Schwartz, M.S. (1983) Iatrogenic neuromuscular disorders: a review. *J. Roy. Soc. Med.*, **76**, 1414–1451.

Swash, M. and Schwartz, M.S. (1988) *Neuromuscular Diseases: A Practical Approach to Diagnosis and Management*, 2nd edn, Springer-Verlag, London.

Thornell, L.-E., Edstrom, L., Eriksson, A. *et al.* (1980) The distribution of intermediate filament protein (skeletin) in normal and diseased human skeletal muscle. *J. Neurol. Sci.*, **47**, 153–620.
Warszanski, M., Telerman-Toppet, N., Durdu, J. *et al.* (1975) The early stages of neuromuscular regeneration after crushing the sciatic nerve in the rat. *J. Neurol. Sci.*, **24**, 21–32.
Webb, J.N. (1977) Cell death in developing skeletal muscle: histochemistry and ultrastructure. *J. Pathol.*, **123**, 175–180.
Willison, R.G. (1980) Arrangement of muscle fibres of a single motor unit in mammalian muscle. *Muscle Nerve*, **3**, 360–361.
Wohlfart, G. (1957) Collateral regeneration from residual motor nerve fibres in amyotrophic lateral sclerosis. *Neurology (Minneap.)*, **7**, 124–134.
Wohlfart, G. (1958) Collateral regeneration in partially denervated muscle. *Neurology (Minneap.)*, **8**, 175–180.
Zenker, F.A. (1864) Ueber die Veränderungen der Willkurlichen Muskeln im Thyphus abdominalis. Vogel, Leipzig.

5 Inflammatory myopathies

Inflammatory myopathy is a common and complex problem in the muscle laboratory. Although these disorders are relatively uncommon in clinical practice, in our experience this is the presumptive diagnosis in nearly half the muscle biopsies sent to the laboratory. Accurate diagnosis of inflammatory myopathies is particularly important not only because treatment is possible, but because the unwanted effects of this treatment cannot lightly be disregarded.

There are a number of different varieties of inflammatory myopathy (Table 5.1). This classification is based on clinical associations (see

Table 5.1 Classification of inflammatory myopathies

Idiopathic polymyositis
Idiopathic dermatomyositis
Childhood-type dermatomyositis
Inclusion body polymyositis

Dermatomyositis or polymyositis associated with autoimmune disorders
  (a) Polyarteritis nodosa
  (b) Rheumatoid arthritis
  (c) Systemic lupus erythematosus
  (d) Scleroderma
  (e) Mixed connective tissue disease
  (f) Polymyositis associated with myasthenia gravis
  (g) Graft vs host myositis
  (h) Penicillamine-induced polymyositis

Sarcoid myopathy

Related conditions
  (a) Polymyalgia rheumatica and giant-cell arteritis
  (b) Eosinophilic fasciitis and myositis

Polymyositis due to infections
  (a) Viral and postinfection myositis, including retrovirus infections
  (b) Bacterial myositis
  (c) Infestations of muscle

Whitaker, 1982; Plotz *et al.*, 1989). However, in all these disorders the pathological features of inflammatory myopathy are found in the muscle biopsy. In some, for example sarcoid myopathy, or in infestations of muscle, e.g. trichinosis, certain additional specific features may be recognized, but the underlying inflammatory myopathy is the cornerstone of the diagnosis. Polymyalgia rheumatica, giant-cell arteritis and eosinophilic fasciitis are inflammatory disorders involving vessels or fascia that although related to myositis are not associated with inflammatory destruction of muscle fibres.

5.1   Clinical features of inflammatory myopathies

The disorder may present acutely or subacutely with painful and weak muscles, usually affecting proximal muscles more than distal but not necessarily symmetrically. Arthralgia, Raynaud's phenomenon, dysphagia, fever, lethargy, anorexia and weight loss are common features. In patients with dermatomyositis there is cutaneous involvement consisting of a characteristic, violaceous, photosensitive skin rash affecting the upper eyelids, cheeks, nose, knuckles, elbows and knees. The rash may precede or accompany muscular symptoms. The skin later becomes shiny and atrophic and the nail beds reddened. In some patients telangiectasia and nail-bed infarcts, a feature of vasculitis, develop. Women are more commonly affected than men, with a peak incidence in the 5th decade. In clinical practice a distinction is drawn between polymyositis and dermatomyositis not only on the basis of cutaneous involvement in the latter disorder but also because of the features noted in Table 5.2. Inclusion body myositis is a disorder that forms a subgroup of idiopathic inflammatory myopathy in which there are no features of

Table 5.2   Clinical features of adult-onset polymyositis and dermatomyositis (from Karpati and Carpenter, 1988)

	Polymyositis	*Dermatomyositis*
Male : female ratio	1 : 1	1 : 2
Distribution of weakness	Proximal	Proximal
Respiratory muscle weakness	—	May be prominent
Dysphagia	Rare	Common
Skin rash	—	Present
Evolution of illness	Chronic	Acute/subacute
Raynaud's phenomenon	Frequent	Rare
Involvement of lung and heart	Rare	Common
Association with carcinoma	Not associated	About 20%

involvement of tissues other than muscle, and in which there are characteristic changes in the muscle biopsy.

In autoimmune disorders, polymyositis may be a presenting feature or, more commonly, a later development in the natural history of the disease. As a rule polymyositis in patients with rheumatoid arthritis, scleroderma, and systemic lupus erythematosus is relatively mild, but it may be more severe in polyarteritis nodosa. Symptoms usually outweigh pathological changes in muscle biopsies in polymyalgia rheumatica and giant-cell arteritis. Sarcoid myopathy is an uncommon disorder usually more marked by pathological change than by symptoms. In childhood-type dermatomyositis muscle contractures are common; a viral infection may precede the muscular syndrome in 25% of children. Muscle pain is severe, but involvement of other organs is uncommon and there is no association with cancer.

5.2   Laboratory investigations

The creatine kinase (CK) is raised in most cases at diagnosis, and the ESR is increased in about half the cases. Other muscle enzymes can be detected in the blood, e.g. aldolase and pyruvate kinase. In severe, active cases myoglobinuria can be demonstrated. Tests for the detection of autoimmune disorders such as autoantibody titres, ESR, antinuclear factor and latex fixation tests, and plasma protein electrophoresis are most helpful in patients with recognized autoimmune syndromes such as rheumatoid arthritis or systemic lupus erythematosus, but they may also show abnormalities in patients with polymyositis, particularly if there are features of mixed connective tissue disease. The ECG is abnormal in some patients but symptomatic cardiomyopathy is relatively uncommon. Investigations for occult neoplasms are generally unrewarding in patients under the age of 40 years without skin involvement. Pulmonary interstitial fibrosis may occur, and is associated with anti-JO-1, myositis-specific circulating autoantibodies.

5.3   Pathology

The changes found in muscle biopsies vary according to the severity and duration of the disease, and the effect of treatment, if any. Particularly characteristic abnormalities occur in the early stages of the illness (Table 5.3). Selection of an appropriately involved muscle for biopsy is particularly important in inflammatory myopathies. The cellular infiltration consists of both B and T cells, including T-cytotoxic and T-killer cells. Studies of the nature of the cellular infiltrate have not revealed features relevant to prognosis or treatment.

Table 5.3 Histological features of idiopathic inflammatory myopathies

Endomysial and interfascicular inflammatory cell infiltration
Single-fibre necrosis with phagocytosis
Basophilic regenerating fibres
Focal distribution of abnormalities in the biopsy
Intrafascicular infarction
Perifascicular fibre atrophy
Moth-eaten fibres
Other myopathic features

5.3.1 *Idiopathic polymyositis*

Inflammatory cell infiltrates are a major feature of most cases and are an important clue to diagnosis. They consist of aggregates of small lymphocytes together with macrophages, plasma cells, and occasionally eosinophils. These cellular infiltrates occur mainly within fascicles in relation to necrotic fibres (Fig. 5.1) or to some small intrafascicular blood vessels (Fig. 5.2). In some biopsies focal cellular infiltrates are not found but in these cases there may be a diffuse increase in cellularity in the endomysium (Fig. 5.3). A diffuse increase in cellularity is also a feature of

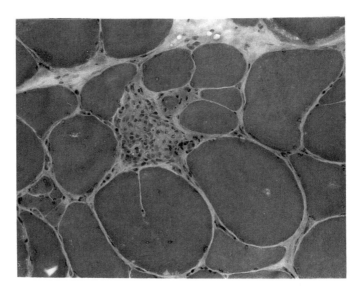

Fig. 5.1 Adult-onset polymyositis × 180; HE. There is an isolated necrotic fibre containing macrophages and a sparse, closely related inflammatory cell response nearby. There is a split fibre, and marked variability in fibre size.

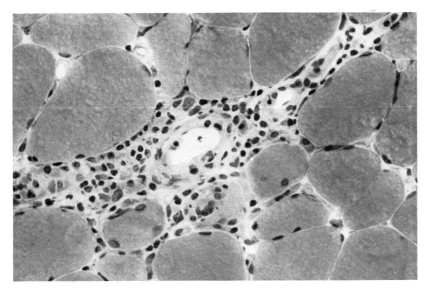

Fig. 5.2 × 350; HE. Acute polymyositis in an adult. The blood vessel is surrounded by lymphocytes and by a few plasma cells. The necrotic fibre is pale and contains macrophages. Several neighbouring fibres are smaller than normal and show enlarged, centrally placed nuclei. These fibres are faintly basophilic, suggesting active regeneration.

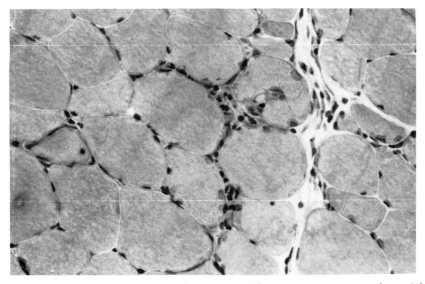

Fig. 5.3 × 350; HE. Acute polymyositis. There is a sparse endomysial lymphocytic infiltrate varying in intensity in different parts of the biopsy. One fibre shows a necrotic segment.

acute toxic myopathies in which muscle fibre necrosis has occurred, and focal inflammatory cell exudates may be a feature of some cases of facioscapulohumeral muscular dystrophy. They are therefore not absolutely diagnostic of inflammatory autoimmune polymyositis. Thrombosis and vasculitis are not commonly seen, but when present are often focal. Fibrinoid necrosis of small vessels is very uncommon. Sometimes perivascular inflammatory cell infiltrates seem to be located near small veins rather than arterioles, a feature particularly found in the rare form of vasculitis described by Churg and Strauss (1951). Endomysial and interfascicular fibrosis, and areas of fat replacement, are features only of chronic polymyositis.

Scattered necrotic muscle fibres, occurring singly or in small clusters, with or without an active macrophage response, are a characteristic feature. They are frequently pale and 'ghost-like' in morphology. These abnormal fibres often show histological features of regeneration, especially basophilia. Scattered atrophic fibres are common and there is usually increased central nucleation.

In up to a quarter of muscle biopsies from patients with the clinical syndrome of idiopathic polymyositis, inflammatory cell infiltrates are

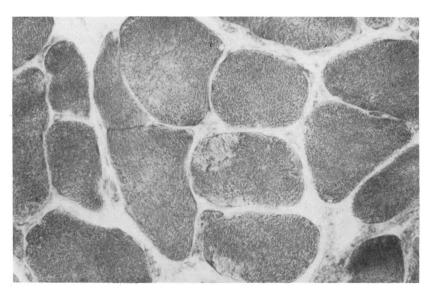

Fig. 5.4 × 350; NADH. Polymyositis. Several fibres show a moth-eaten appearance consisting of patchy areas of absent enzyme activity. Note the variability in fibre size and the separation of the fibres, caused by thickening of the interstitial tissue.

absent. In these cases the diagnosis should be corsidered on the basis of the other histological features, especially the occurrence of active degeneration and regeneration, moth-eaten fibres (Fig. 5.4) and the focal distribution of the abnormality.

5.3.2 Chronic idiopathic polymyositis

The histopathology of chronic polymyositis is summarized in Table 5.4. The main differences between chronic and acute polymyositis are the features of relatively chronic myopathic change (Fig. 5.5), consisting of marked variation in fibre size with hypertrophied fibres, fibre splitting, central nucleation, regenerating fibres and fibrosis (Fig. 5.6). These changes may resemble those of a limb-girdle dystrophy (Fig. 5.7). However, the diagnosis of chronic polymyositis is suggested by the endomysial inflammatory cell infiltrate (Fig. 5.8) with the myopathic features (Swash and Schwartz, 1977). Further, architectural changes are often very prominent in chronic polymyositis and these histological abnormalities are usually focally distributed within the biopsy, whereas in muscular dystrophies the abnormalities are diffusely distributed.

In some biopsies small groups of muscle fibres of the same histochemical type may be noted; in combination with the other histological features this is a characteristic finding. The presence of marked focal inflammatory cell aggregates in a biopsy showing the features of the chronic stage of the disease suggests continuing disease activity, or relapse. In advanced polymyositis, when there has been severe loss of muscle fibres, the biopsy contains islands of abnormal muscle fibres in zones of fatty and fibrous connective tissue. At this late stage of the disease the histological appearances may be non-specific, and

Table 5.4 Histological features of chronic idiopathic polymyositis

Myopathic features:
   Marked variation in fibre size
   Hypertrophied fibres
   Central nucleation
   Fibre splitting
   Regenerating and necrotic fibres
   Endomysial and perifascicular fibrosis
Prominent architectural changes in individual fibres, often focally distributed
Inflammatory cell exudates

Neurogenic features:
   Fibre-type grouping (usually not prominent)
   Scattered atrophic, pointed, NADH-dark fibres

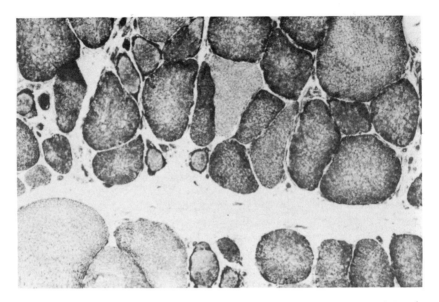

Fig. 5.5 × 140; NADH. Chronic polymyositis. There is marked variability in fibre size and in the intensity of the enzyme reactivity. Several smaller fibres show increased enzyme reactivity in their rims. Minor moth-eaten architectural changes in the NADH reaction are present. These are non-specific myopathic features. The interfascicular plane is thickened.

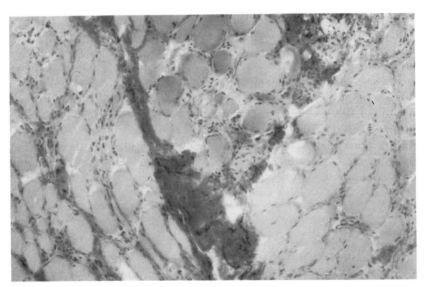

Fig. 5.6 × 140; Van-Gieson stain. Chronic polymyositis. Sheets of fibrous tissue separate the fascicles and, in some parts of the biopsy, interstitial fibrosis is also prominent. There is a sparse patchy cellular infiltrate mainly in relation to necrotic fibres.

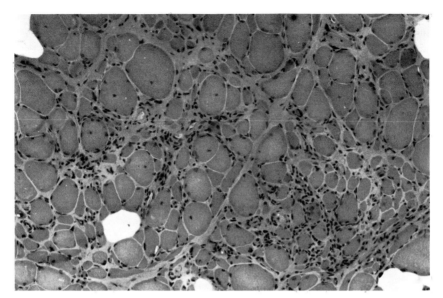

Fig. 5.7 × 140; HE. Chronic active polymyositis. There is marked variation in fibre size with endomysial fibrosis. Many small fibres are present. The disease is active, as shown by the prominent focal lymphocytic aggregates. The appearance resembles that of limb-girdle muscular dystrophy.

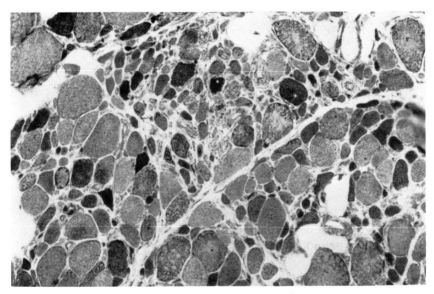

Fig. 5.8 × 140; NADH. Chronic active polymyositis. In this section, adjacent to Fig. 5.7, the variable enzyme reactivity of large and small fibres can be seen, showing the diversity of the morphological changes in individual fibres in this disease.

similar abnormalities may be found in dystrophies and chronic neurogenic disorders. It is thus important that the biopsy be taken from moderately or mildly affected muscles, rather than from very atrophic muscles.

Type 2 fibre atrophy is frequently found in biopsies in chronic polymyositis. This is particularly prominent in patients treated with steroids, but may also develop as a result of disuse. Secondary steroid myopathy may be suspected when the biopsy shows prominent neutral lipid droplets in Type 1 muscle fibres.

5.3.3   Dermatomyositis in adults and children

The clinical features are summarized in Table 5.2. The major feature is the association of a rash with the muscle disease. In general, dermatomyositis is a more serious illness than polymyositis, with more severe weakness and greater morbidity and mortality, especially from the development of interstitial lung disease and cardiomyopathy. Dermatomyositis represents about a third of all cases of inflammatory myopathy. About 20% of adult-onset cases of dermatomyositis are associated with cancer.

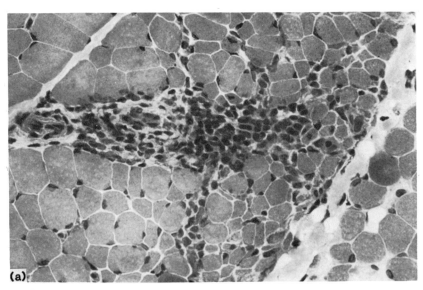

(a)

Fig. 5.9 Childhood dermatomyositis, × 350; HE. A prominent focal lymphocytic infiltrate is situated in a muscle fascicle in relation to a thickened blood vessel (at the left edge of the illustration). Perifascicular atrophy is prominent but an adjoining fascicle (right) contains fibres of normal size.

This association is stronger in older patients, especially for cancers of the lung and gastrointestinal tract in men, and of the breast and ovary in women (Callen, 1984).

The histological features of adult dermatomyositis differ in many respects from those of myositis without cutaneous involvement. Although the histological hallmark of both conditions is inflammation, the distribution of the inflammatory infiltrates differs. In dermatomyositis the inflammatory cell infiltrates tend to be perivascular or in the interfascicular septa rather than within the fascicles (Fig. 5.9). *Muscle infarction* is a particular feature of dermatomyositis. This is associated with necrosis of arterioles and capillaries. Electron microscopy reveals undulated tubules in the endothelial cells of muscle capillaries. These cells are often surrounded by a reduplicated basal lamina, suggesting that they have previously undergone regeneration (Banker, 1975). Deposition of IgG and complement has been reported in small

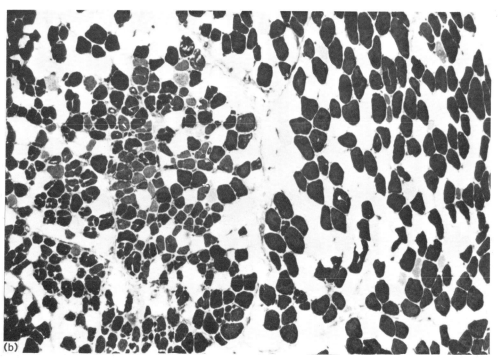

(b)

Fig. 5.10   Adult-onset dermatomyositis. × 60. ATPase pH 4.3. A zone of regenerating small fibres (to the left of the illustration) occupies several fascicles, suggesting a vascular basis for fibre necrosis.

blood vessels in muscle biopsies of dermatomyositis (Whitaker and Engel, 1972; Kissel *et al.*, 1986). Muscle infarction may involve groups of muscle fibres, or even part of a fascicle (Fig. 5.10). There is usually a marked loss of capillaries in these regions (Banker, 1975; Carpenter *et al.*, 1976). All the fibres involved in these microinfarcts thus appear to be at the same stage of necrosis or regeneration (Fig. 5.10). *Perifascicular atrophy* is a characteristic feature, consisting of atrophic fibres at the periphery of the fascicle. Many of these abnormal fibres are rounded, and show architectural change (Figs 5.9, 5.11), an appearance that is thought to be due to ischaemia of the periphery of affected fascicles. Moth-eaten fibres may be prominent in the biopsy (Fig. 5.11) and necrosis, phagocytosis and regenerating fibres are frequently seen. In clinically severe cases, endomysial oedema is often a feature. In the childhood-onset form of dermatomyositis (Banker and Victor, 1966) the histological appearances are similar to those of acute adult-onset dermatomyositis. Perifascicular atrophy is often particularly prominent (Fig. 5.11).

Skin biopsies may also be helpful in making the diagnosis. The erythematous lesions show changes resembling those found in systemic lupus erythematosus. Epidermal atrophy with oedema of the upper dermis, degeneration of the basal cell layers and a scattered inflammatory cell infiltrate, or features of vasculitis, may be seen. Focal panniculitis of the subcutaneous tissue layers is also a common feature, and calcification may be present.

5.3.4   Inclusion body myositis (IBM)

IBM is a form of inflammatory myopathy (Carpenter *et al.*, 1978) without cutaneous involvement, with a 3 : 1 male predominance, insidious onset after the age of 50 years, proximal and distal weakness and a normal or only mildly raised blood CK level. There is a weak association with diabetes mellitus, autoimmune disease, and peripheral neuropathy (Lotz *et al.*, 1989). The condition is characterized histologically by the presence of rimmed vacuoles in the biopsy. These are often sparse, occurring only with a frequency of one per low-power field. Inflammatory-cell infiltration is found in the endomysium and in relation to blood vessels in most cases, and atrophic or necrotic fibres are common. Eosinophilic inclusions may be present in some muscle fibres. Rimmed vacuoles consist of irregular vacuoles 2–25 μm in diameter, lined or rimmed by basophilic granular material that may also be found within the vacuoles and that stains positively also in Sudan black B and acid haematoxylin preparations. These vacuoles are usually negative for acid phosphatase. There is no fibre-type predilection. These vacuoles have mostly been reported in the gastrocnemius muscle (Carpenter and Karpati, 1984).

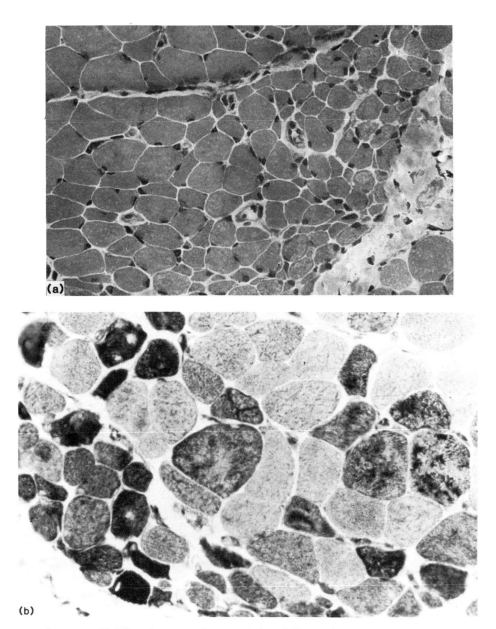

Fig. 5.11 Childhood-onset polymyositis (aged 15 years).
(a) × 350; HE. Perifascicular atrophy, interfascicular fibrosis and mild architectural changes, especially in the perifascicular region, are the main abnormalities. In this section, inflammatory cell exudates are not a feature.
(b)× 617; NADH. There are prominent architectural changes, with moth-eaten fibres and perifascicular atrophy.

Electron microscopy reveals intracytoplasmic and intranuclear filamentous inclusions 10–20 nm in diameter. The vacuoles are filled with
cytoplasmic degradation products, thus resembling autophagic vacuoles.
IBM is a disorder of unknown aetiology that does not respond to steroid
therapy and that progresses inexorably. Rimmed vacuoles and filamentous inclusions may also occur in distal myopathies, and oculopharyngeal dystrophy.

5.4   Muscle involvement in other autoimmune disorders

Inflammatory myopathy may complicate other autoimmune diseases,
and there are some differences in the histological features of the
myopathy found in these conditions.

5.4.1   Polyarteritis nodosa

In this disease the typical features of polymyositis may be found,
accompanied by prominent vasculitis, often affecting arterioles, small
arteries or veins. The media is most often affected and may become
necrotic and eosinophilic. Necrosis extends into the intima leading to
thrombus formation within the lumen of the vessel. The internal elastic
lamina is almost always involved. Neutrophils and eosinophils are
characteristic of the early vascular lesion, but later, lymphocytes, plasma
cells and macrophages predominate. At this stage the affected vessels
become thickened and nodular. The muscle lesions in polyarteritis
nodosa are due to infarction, but haemorrhage may also occur. The
lesions vary in age and severity in different parts of the muscle.

Polyarteritis nodosa involves both nerve and muscle (Fig. 5.12).
Histological features of denervation, i.e. small, angular, NADH-dark
fibres, or of reinnervation, i.e. fibre-type grouping, are characteristic in
muscle biopsies in this disorder. At least 30% of patients with
polyarteritis nodosa show clinical signs of involvement of muscle;
however, muscle biopsy is probably less useful in the diagnosis of this
condition than has been suggested in the past (Wallace *et al.*, 1958).

5.4.2   Rheumatoid arthritis

Involvement of muscle is common in rheumatoid arthritis, but active
polymyositis is relatively uncommon (Pitkeathley and Coomes, 1966).
Type 2 atrophy occurs in muscles relatively immobilized by joint disease,
and moth-eaten and whorled fibres may be found. Later, in more
advanced cases, atrophy of both fibre types occurs. An inflammatory
response in the endomysium and interfascicular tissue, without muscle

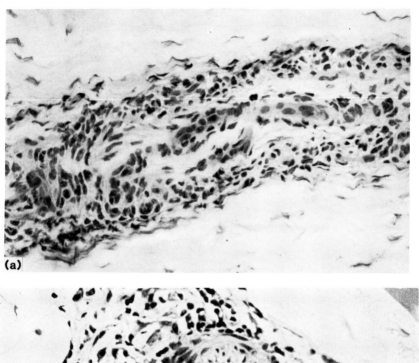

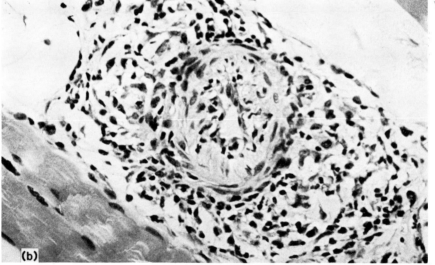

Fig. 5.12 × 350; HE. Polyarteritis nodosa. (a) Sural nerve biopsy; the endoneurial blood vessel, sectioned obliquely, shows lymphocytic infiltration. (b) Cellular infiltration around a thickened small artery in a muscle biopsy.

fibre necrosis or vasculitis, is a common feature of rheumatoid arthritis, occurring in about half the cases (Dubowitz, 1985; Haslock *et al.*, 1970).

Disturbances of the innervation of muscle are common in rheumatoid arthritis due to symmetrical polyneuropathy, root lesions or mononeuritis multiplex, especially in patients with rheumatoid vasculitis, and these complications may lead to neurogenic changes in affected muscles, especially in distal muscles.

5.4.3 Systemic lupus erythematosus

Polymyositis is infrequent in systemic lupus, occurring in only 3% of patients in one series (Ester and Christian, 1971). Individual fibres sometimes show vacuoles in association with central nuclei. Although vasculitis is a feature of the disease, hyaline thickening, fibrinoid necrosis or thrombotic occlusion of intramuscular blood vessels is uncommon in muscle biopsies (see Fig. 5.13). A sparse lymphocytic endomysial infiltration may be a feature.

5.4.4   Scleroderma (progressive systemic sclerosis)

Muscular stiffness is common but active polymyositis is a rare complication of this disorder. There are no specific histological features of

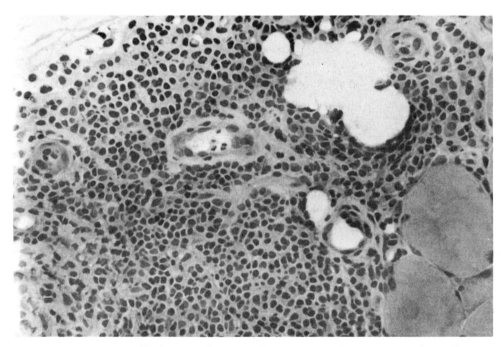

Fig. 5.13   × 427; HE. Systemic lupus erythematosus. A dense mononuclear cell infiltrate surrounds a small blood vessel, the wall of which is thickened.

this complication. Muscle biopsies in uncomplicated scleroderma reveal little or no abnormality.

5.4.5   *Mixed connective tissue disease*

This is a clinical syndrome in which features of various autoimmune disorders coexist. Muscle biopsies often reveal a diffuse but sparse inflammatory cell exudate, but fibre necrosis or regeneration are relatively uncommon features. In some cases, perivascular inflammatory cell exudates may occur.

5.4.6   *Sarcoid myopathy*

Although sarcoidosis of muscle may be found coincidentally or on muscle biopsy in about 30% of all cases of systemic sarcoidosis, clinically evident sarcoid myopathy is uncommon. The muscle biopsy shows typical sarcoid granulomata, or infiltration with small epithelioid cells (Fig. 5.14). Muscle fibre destruction occurs in the region of the granulomata but isolated degenerating or regenerating muscle fibres are not a feature.

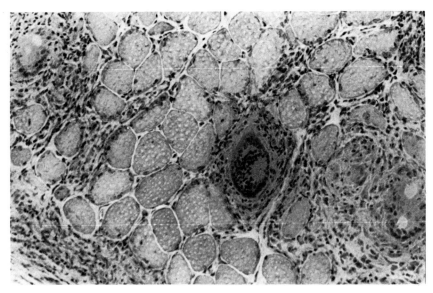

Fig. 5.14   × 140; HE. Sarcoidosis. A granuloma accompanied by an intense lymphocytic cellular infiltrate within the muscle. The multinuclear giant cell was not associated with acid-fast bacilli, and the diagnosis of sarcoidosis was confirmed by clinical investigation.

5.4.7   Polymyalgia rheumatica

In this disorder muscle stiffness at rest, relieved by activity, is accompanied by fever, malaise and a raised ESR. Most cases occur in women over 55 years of age; there is an association with *temporal arteritis*. The muscle biopsy shows Type 2B fibre atrophy with occasional moth-eaten and whorled fibres. Inflammatory cell infiltrates and increased central nucleation are *not* features of this disorder. These changes resemble those found in mild cases of rheumatoid arthritis.

5.4.8   Eosinophilic fasciitis

Clinically this rare disorder may resemble idiopathic polymyositis. The muscle biopsy reveals large numbers of round cells in the fascial planes, with moderate numbers of eosinophils (Fig. 5.15). The muscle shows only mild structural changes (Nassanova *et al.*, 1979) but these may resemble polymyositis in some cases (Stark, 1979).

5.4.9   Eosinophilic polymyositis

Hypereosinophilia, detected in peripheral blood, may be associated with

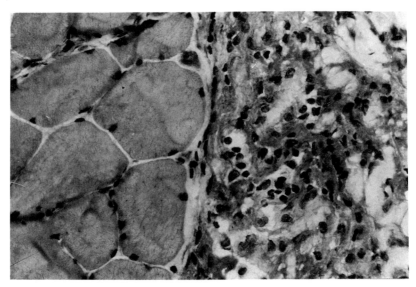

Fig. 5.15   Eosinophilic fasciitis. × 350; HE. There is an infiltrate of small round cells in the fascia at the superficial margin of the muscle. In this condition there is an eosinophilia in the blood. The muscle itself is normal, or shows only minor abnormalities.

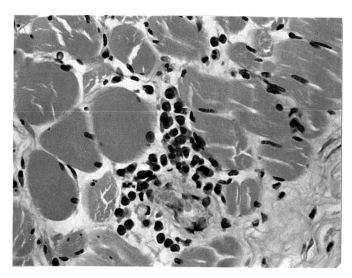

Fig. 5.16   Eosinophilic polymyositis. HE. × 360. Paraffin-embedded tissue. Cellular infiltrate consisting virtually entirely of eosinophils. There is increased variability in fibre size.

myositis and an eosinophilic infiltrate in the affected muscle (Fig. 5.16). There are three clinical syndromes. Eosinophilic polymyositis is a systemic disease (Layzer *et al.*, 1977) in which hypereosinophilia and myositis are associated with a rash, subcutaneous oedema, pulmonary infiltrates and peripheral neuropathy. This syndrome has a poor prognosis. In focal eosinophilic myositis there are focal eosinophilic muscle infiltrates without muscular weakness or systemic features. In eosinophilic perimyositis the inflammation is perimysial, there is no systemic involvement and the course is benign (Lakhanpal *et al.*, 1988).

5.4.10   Infestations of muscle

A variety of parasites have been reported as invading skeletal muscle (Pallis and Lewis, 1981) but infestation of muscle is a rare clinical finding in the United Kingdom, and in other developed countries. Only cysticercosis (*Taenia solium*), trichinosis (*Trichinella spiralis*) and toxocariasis (*Toxocara canis*) are at all likely to be found in muscle biopsies. In trichinosis (Fig. 5.17) the parasite is found inside muscle fibres of either histochemical type leading to muscle-fibre necrosis, with an intense eosinophilic and macrophage cellular response. In cysticercosis the cysts consist of multiple vesicles surrounded by a mild inflammatory cell exudate in which eosinophils may be prominent. In the late stages these

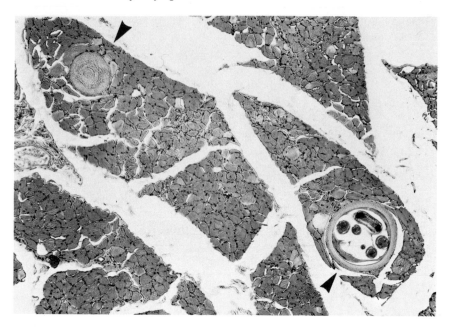

Fig. 5.17   × 100; paraffin-embedded, HE. Trichinosis of muscle. Two spiral parasites, firmly encased, without reactive cellular response, can be seen (arrows). This represents the chronic, inactive stage of the disease. (Illustration kindly supplied by Dr Uros Roessman, University Hospitals of Cleveland, Ohio, USA.)

cysts form calcified nodules. Other organs are almost invariably involved. Toxocariasis has been recognized relatively recently as an infestation of children.

5.4.11   Infections of muscle

Occasionally fungal infection may occur, particularly in patients with overwhelming fungal septicaemia. Bacterial abscesses in muscles develop from contiguous spread from neighbouring infections, e.g. osteomyelitis or cutaneous ulcers, or from haematogenous invasion. Tuberculosis of muscle is very rare. Syphilitic granulomata are also very uncommon.

5.4.12   Myasthenia gravis

Muscle biopsies are not usually performed in the investigation of myasthenia gravis unless there is suspicion of coincidental polymyositis, or a metabolic myopathy, for example hyperthyroid myopathy. Polymyositis and myasthenia gravis may occur in the same patient either at the same time or separately (Johns *et al.*, 1971).

In myasthenia gravis the commonest abnormality is Type 2 fibre atrophy; this was found in about half the biopsies reported by Engel and McFarlin (1966). Type 2 fibre atrophy is not always uniformly distributed, even appearing focally in the biopsy (Dubowitz, 1985). Lymphocytic infiltrates, first described by Buzzard (1905) as 'lymphorrhages', consisting of aggregates of lymphocytes situated in the endomysium, unrelated to blood vessels (Russell, 1953), are found in about a quarter of cases biopsied, but are found more commonly at autopsy. Histological features of denervation, consisting of clusters of small, pointed fibres of either histochemical type, or features of reinnervation, e.g. fibre-type grouping, occur in some cases, particularly those in whom the disease has been severe and of considerable duration (Brownell *et al.*, 1972). The motor end-plates show characteristic histological abnormalities by both light and electron microscopy (Coërs *et al.*, 1973), consisting of expanded, proliferated endings, or elongated endings lacking side branches. In addition, there is often increased collateral sprouting at the terminal arborization of the end-plate. Whilst these changes are mainly due to the disease, they may be due, in part, to the effects of long-term anticholinesterase therapy (Schwartz *et al.*, 1977).

Myasthenia gravis is a disorder of neuromuscular transmission in which the α subunit of the acetylcholine receptor protein in the motor end-plate is blocked and degraded by a complement-mediated reaction with a circulating antibody in the IgG compartment. The abnormality is thus postsynaptic and IgG and C3 are deposited at this site (Engel *et al.*, 1977). The postjunctional end-plate membrane is disrupted and the synaptic cleft widened and simplified. This antigen–antibody reaction is accompanied by a local macrophage response and by morphological changes and physiological abnormalities in the motor end-plate which account for the clinical and pathological features of the disease (see Albuquerque *et al.*, 1976 and Swash and Schwartz, 1988 for reviews).

Thymomas are found in 10% of patients with myasthenia gravis; in the remainder the thymus shows hyperplasia, or may be normal.

References

Albuquerque, E.X., Rash, J.E., Mayer, R.F. and Satterfield, R. (1976) Electrophysiological and morphological study of the neuromuscular function in patients with myasthenia gravis. *Exp. Neurol.*, **51**, 536–563.
Banker, B.Q. (1975) Dermatomyositis of childhood: ultrastructural alteration of muscle and intramuscular blood vessels. *J. Neuropathol. Exp. Neurol.*, **34**, 46–75.

104   Inflammatory myopathies

Banker, B.Q. and Victor, M. (1966) Dermatomyositis (systemic angiopathy) of childhood. *Medicine (Balt.)*, **45**, 261–289.

Brownell, B., Oppenheimer, J.R. and Spalding, J.M.K. (1972) Neurogenic muscle atrophy in myasthenia gravis. *J. Neurol. Neurosurg. Psychiatry*, **34**, 311–322.

Buzzard, E.F. (1905) The clinical history and post mortem examination in five cases of myasthenia gravis. *Brain*, **28**, 438–483.

Callen, J.P. (1984) Myositis and malignancy. *Clin. Rheum. Dis.*, **10**, 117–130.

Carpenter, S. and Karpati, G. (1984) *Pathology of Skeletal Muscle*, Churchill Livingstone, New York, pp. 754.

Carpenter, S., Karpati, G., Heller, I. and Eisen, A. (1978) Inclusion body myositis: a distinct variety of idiopathic inflammatory myopathy. *Neurology*, **28**, 8–17.

Carpenter, S., Karpati, G., Rothman, S. and Watters, G. (1976) The childhood type of dermatomyositis. *Neurology*, **26**, 952–962.

Churg, J. and Strauss, L. (1951) Allergic granulomatosis, allergic angiitis and periarteritis nodosa. *Am. J. Pathol.*, **27**, 277–302.

Coërs, C., Tellerman-Toppet, N. and Gerard, J.-M. (1973) Terminal innervation ratio in neuromuscular disease: disorders of lower motor neuron, peripheral nerve and muscle. *Arch. Neurol.*, **29**, 215–222.

Dubowitz, V. (1985) *Muscle Biopsy – A Practical Approach*, W.B. Saunders, London, pp. 720.

Engel, A.G., Lambert, E.H. and Howard, F.M. Jr. (1977) Immune complexes (IgC & C₃) at the motor end plate in myasthenia gravis. *Mayo Clin. Proc.*, **52**, 267–280.

Engel, W.K. and McFarlin, D.E. (1966) Discussion of paper by Fenichel. *Ann. NY Acad. Sci.*, **135**, 68-77.

Ester, D. and Christian, C.L. (1971) The natural history of systemic lupus erythematosus by prospective analysis. *Medicine (Balt.)*, **50**, 85–95.

Haslock, D.I., Wright, V. and Harriman, D.G.F. (1970) Neuromuscular disorders in rheumatoid arthritis: a motor point muscle biopsy study. *Q.J. Med.*, **39**, 335–358.

Johns, T.R., Crowley, W.J., Miller, J.Q. and Campa, J.F. (1971) The syndrome of myasthenia and polymyositis, with comments on therapy. *Ann. NY Acad. Sci.*, **183**, 64–71.

Karpati, G. and Carpenter, S. (1988) Idiopathic inflammatory myopathies. *Curr. Opin. Neurol. Neurosurg.*, **1**, 806–814.

Kissel, J.T., Mendell, J.R. and Rammohan, K.W. (1986) Microvascular deposition of complement membrane attack complex in dermatomyositis. *N. Engl. J. Med.*, **314**, 329–334.

Lakhanpal, S., Duffy, J. and Engel, A.G. (1988) Eosinophilia associated with perimyositis and pneumonitis. *Mayo Clin. Proc.*, **63**, 37–41.

Layzer, R.B., Shearn, M.A. and Satyamurti, S. (1977) Eosinophilic polymyositis. *Ann. Neurol.*, **1**, 65–71.

Lotz, B.P., Engel, A.G., Nishino, H. *et al.* (1989) Inclusion body myositis. *Brain*, **112**, 727–747.

Nassanova, V.A., Ivanova, M.M., Akhnazarova, V.D. *et al.* (1979) Eosinophilic fasciitis. *Scand. J. Rheum.*, **8**, 225–233.

Pallis, C. and Lewis, P.D. (1981) Inflammatory myopathies: involvement of human muscle by parasites. In *Disorders of Voluntary Muscle*, 4th edn (ed. J.N. Walton), Churchill Livingstone, Edinburgh, pp. 569–584.

Pitkeathley, D.A. and Coomes, E.N. (1966) Polymyositis in rheumatoid arthritis. *Ann. Rheum. Dis.*, **25**, 127–132.

Plotz, P.H., Dalakas, M.C., Left, R.L. *et al.* (1989) Current concepts in the idiopathic inflammatory myopathies: polymyositis, dermatomyositis and related disorders. *Ann. Intern. Med.*, **111**, 143–157.

Russell, D.S. (1953) Histological changes in the striped muscles in myasthenia gravis. *J. Pathol.*, **65**, 279–289.

Schwartz, M.S., Sargeant, M.K. and Swash, M. (1977) Neostigmine-induced end plate proliferation in the rat. *Neurology*, **27**, 289–293.

Stark, R.J. (1979) Eosinophilic polymyositis. *Arch. Neurol.*, **36**, 721–722.

Swash, M. and Schwartz, M.S. (1977) Implications of longitudinal muscle fibre splitting in neurogenic and myopathic disorders. *J. Neurol. Neurosurg. Psychiatry*, **40**, 1152–1159.

Swash, M. and Schwartz, M.S. (1988) *Neuromuscular Diseases: A Practical Approach to Diagnosis and Management* (2nd edn), Springer-Verlag, Berlin, pp. 456.

Wallace, S.L., Lattis, R. and Ragan, C. (1958) Diagnostic significance of the muscle biopsy. *Am. J. Med.*, **25**, 600–610.

Whitaker, J.N. (1982) Inflammatory myopathy: a review of etiologic and pathogenic features. *Muscle Nerve*, **5**, 573–597.

Whitaker, J.N. and Engel, W.K. (1972) Vascular deposits of immunoglobulin and complement in idiopathic inflammatory myopathy. *N. Eng. J. Med.*, **286**, 333–338.

6 Muscular dystrophies

The muscular dystrophies are relatively uncommon inherited disorders of muscle. They are characterized by a progressive course and by degenerative changes in skeletal muscle fibres. Most begin in childhood but in others the disease is not recognized until adult life. Classification depends on clinical, genetic and histological criteria (Table 6.1). The benign childhood myopathies are, by convention, classified separately since these disorders are only very slowly progressive and show only mild myopathic changes in the muscle, although particular diagnostic features occur in certain of these disorders.

6.1 Duchenne muscular dystrophy

This disorder is the most severe form of muscular dystrophy. It is inherited as an X-linked recessive disorder, so that it affects boys only, although cases of affected girls with Turner's syndrome (XO) and with X-autosome balanced translocations have been reported. The trait is carried on the short arm of the X chromosome at the Xp21 locus. The genetic locus is large, a feature that probably accounts for the frequency of the disease and for its high mutation rate. The protein product of the

Table 6.1 Classification of muscular dystrophies

X-linked muscular dystrophies
  Duchenne muscular dystrophy
  Becker muscular dystrophy
  Other X-linked, less severe muscular dystrophies
Scapuloperoneal muscular dystrophy
Limb-girdle muscular dystrophy
Facioscapulohumeral muscular dystrophy
Myotonic dystrophy and other myotonic syndromes
Ocular myopathies
Oculopharyngeal dystrophy

gene, dystrophin, is a 400 kDa protein, comprising only 0.01% of protein in normal muscle cells, that is an essential component of the plasma membrane and of the T tubules (Kunkel and Hoffman, 1989). In affected families in which the mother is known to be a carrier of the gene, half the boys will be affected, and half the girls will be carriers. The disease affects 1 in 3000 male births. It has been estimated that as many as a third of affected boys represent new mutations and in these cases none of the relatives will be carriers. Female carriers may show minor abnormalities, such as hypertrophied calf muscles, slight proximal muscle weakness and, more frequently, a raised CK.

Affected boys always develop the full clinical syndrome. Weakness of girdle muscles, especially pelvic muscles, is apparent before the age of 4 years. Hypertrophy of muscles, especially calves, deltoids and serratus anterior, is an important diagnostic feature. Slight intellectual impairment and an abnormal ECG are often found. The child never runs, and walking is abnormal, with a characteristic waddling, broad-based gait and lordotic posture. Motor milestones are delayed. Most patients lose the ability to walk by the age of 11 years and about 75% die before the age of 21 years. Survival beyond 30 years is unusual (Walton and Gardner-Medwin, 1981).

The CK is greatly raised in all cases, especially in the early stages of the disorder when it may be 20 or more times normal. In female carriers the CK is only slightly raised; in some it may be normal.

6.1.1   Muscle pathology

The changes in muscle biopsies vary according to the stage of the disease (Table 6.2).

The most characteristic histological feature of Duchenne dystrophy is the presence of hyaline fibres (Fig. 6.1); these are especially prominent in the early stages of the disease. They are large rounded fibres which appear homogeneous and vitreous in HE stains. In longitudinal sections the cross-striations are lost. Hyaline fibres stain slightly darker than other fibres, using the HE (Fig. 6.7), Gomori and NADH techniques (Fig. 6.2), and they are a particular feature of the early stage of the disease. Hyaline fibres probably result from hypercontraction of parts of muscle fibres due to uncontrolled entry of calcium into these fibres through the fundamental defect in the plasma membrane. Calcium is concentrated at the edges of these fibres (Fig. 6.3), and this can be demonstrated histologically (Bodensteiner and Engel, 1978). Hyaline change may thus represent the first stage in necrosis of muscle fibres in this disease (Cullen and Fulthorpe, 1975). Walton (1973) noted that in serial sections, adjacent parts of affected fibres are often necrotic and undergoing phagocytosis.

Table 6.2 Sequence of muscle biopsy changes in Duchenne dystrophy

	Early 1–5 years ambulant	Moderately advanced 6–10 years marked weakness	Late 10 years or older chairbound
Hyalinized fibres	———————————	———————————	
Fibre necrosis	———————————	———————————	- - - - - - - - -
Phagocytosis	———————————	———————————	- - - - - - - - -
Fibrosis	- - - - - - - - -	———————————	———————————
Rounded fibres	- - - - - - - - -	———————————	———————————
Regenerating fibres	———————————	———————————	
Central nucleation		———————————	———————————
Fibre splitting		———————————	———————————
Fibre hypertrophy		———————————	———————————
Fat replacement		- - - - - - - - -	———————————
Poor fibre-type differentiation		———————————	———————————

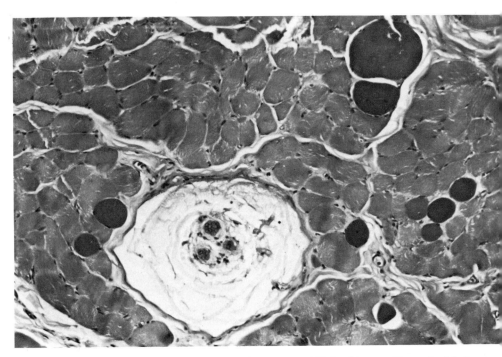

Fig. 6.1 Duchenne muscular dystrophy, × 180; HE. In this paraffin-embedded section a muscle spindle, sectioned through its nuclear bag region, is prominent; its periaxial space is enlarged and contains unusually prominent inner capsular connective tissue. There are fewer than the normal 6–14 intrafusal muscle fibres. In the muscle itself hyaline fibres, which appear dark, rounded and large, are prominent. There is increased endomysial fibrosis.

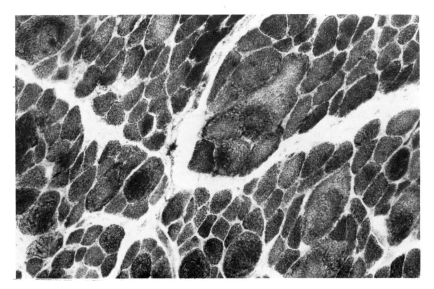

Fig. 6.2 Duchenne muscular dystrophy. × 140; NADH. The fascicles are separated by thickened unstained interfascicular connective tissue. The muscle fibres vary in size and several show zones of increased reactivity. The differentiation of fibre types is less developed than in normal muscle.

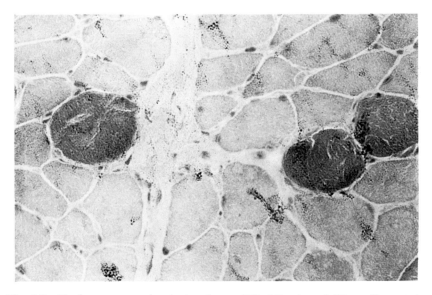

Fig. 6.3 Duchenne muscular dystrophy, × 350; Alizarin red. Three fibres stain intensely, indicating increased calcium content. These are hyaline fibres. Some stain has precipitated on the surface of the section producing areas of dark artefact.

Hyaline fibres are not specific for Duchenne dystrophy since they also occur, although in fewer numbers, in other X-linked dystrophies and, rarely, in limb-girdle dystrophy.

Necrotic fibres undergoing phagocytosis are common in the early and moderately advanced stages of the disease. These are often surrounded by small round cells and macrophages. Clusters of small basophilic regenerating fibres are usually a prominent feature (Fig. 6.4), especially in the earlier stages of the disease. They may be found at any site within a fascicle and they are often associated with an inflammatory cell infiltrate in the endomysium. These fibres usually contain acid phosphatase (Fig. 6.5) as well as sarcoplasmic RNA (Neerunjun and Dubowitz, 1977). The sarcoplasm of these fibres is vesicular and their nuclei contain a dispersed chromatin pattern.

In the middle stages of the disease the muscle fibres appear rounded and show increased variability in size (Fig. 6.6). There is marked interfascicular and endomysial fibrosis even in the early stages when the fascicular pattern is preserved (Fig. 6.7), and the majority of muscle fibres are relatively undamaged. In enzyme histochemical stains fibre-type differentiation is poorly developed in the ATPase preparations so that it may be difficult to distinguish the Type 1 and Type 2 fibres (Fig. 6.6).

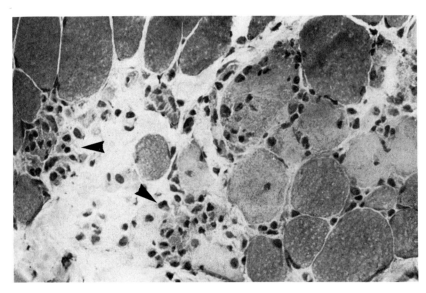

Fig. 6.4 Duchenne muscular dystrophy. × 350; HE. Zones of clustered regenerating fibres (arrows), of varying size and staining characteristics. Some contain central or plump sarcolemmal nuclei, and the fibres vary greatly in size. Some nearby rounded fibres show ice crystal artefact.

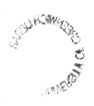

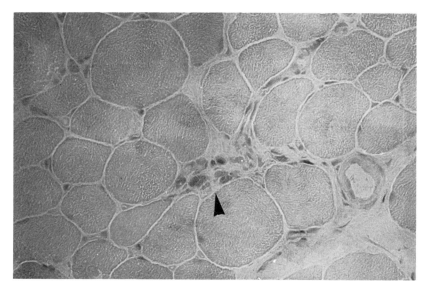

Fig. 6.5 Duchenne muscular dystrophy. × 350; Acid phosphatase. Several small fibres or fibre fragments, associated with necrosis and subsequent regeneration, show a positive reaction (arrow). This is usually associated with lysosomal activity.

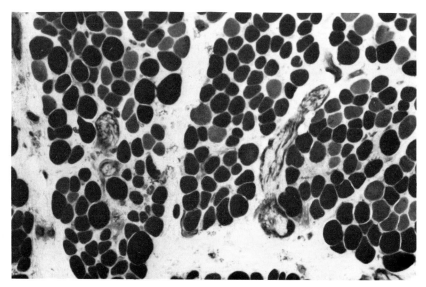

Fig. 6.6 Duchenne muscular dystrophy. × 140; ATPase, pH 4.6. Poor fibre-type differentiation. Note the rounded fibres and their wide separation from each other.

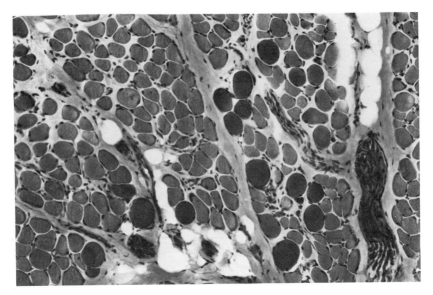

Fig. 6.7 Duchenne muscular dystrophy. × 140; HE. The muscle fibres are all unusually rounded and there are many darkly staining (eosinophilic) hyaline fibres. There is endomysial and interfascicular fibrosis. Adipose tissue is prominent. A nerve bundle appears normal. Several clusters of small atrophic regenerating fibres are present.

When fibre types can be differentiated there is a deficiency of Type 2B fibres but an increased number of Type 2C fibres occurs in most cases. Fibre-type differentiation in the NADH, SDH, glycogen and phosphorylase reactions appear normal, but morphological changes in individual fibres may be demonstrated with these techniques. Both fibre types appear equally involved in these degenerative and regenerative changes (Engel, 1977).

Splitting of muscle fibres may be a prominent feature at a stage of the disease at which the child is still mobile, usually between the ages of 5 and 7 years (Bell and Conen, 1968), but it becomes less prominent later. Muscle fibre hypertrophy is not usually prominent, although the hyaline fibres themselves are larger than the surrounding fibres. The distribution of blood vessels and capillaries in relation to individual muscle fibres is normal. Muscle spindles show thickening of their capsules and enlargement of their periaxial spaces (Fig. 6.1) but are usually relatively well-preserved until the most advanced stage of the disorder (Swash and Fox, 1976). Intramuscular nerve bundles appear normal, even when the muscle is largely destroyed; methylene blue impregnations have shown enlargement of the innervational area of motor end-plates but no collateral sprouting (Coërs and Tellerman-Toppet, 1977).

Electron microscopy is not helpful in diagnosis, but it has been used to demonstrate discontinuities in the plasma membrane of muscle fibres (Mokri and Engel, 1975; Carpenter and Karpati, 1979). The diagnosis can be confirmed by the absence of dystrophin in the muscle fibre membrane, using an affinity-purified anti-dystrophin antibody that detects dystrophin in the plasma membrane of muscle fibres with an immunofluorescent technique (Zubrzycka-Gaarn *et al.*, 1988; Arahata *et al.*, 1989).

6.1.2 *Prenatal diagnosis*

Increased variation in muscle fibre diameter, an increase in the amount of connective tissue and hyalinized fibres have been described in fetuses of 18–20 weeks gestation presumed, on the basis of a family history of the disease and raised placental blood CK levels, to have muscular dystrophy (Emery and Burt, 1980; Mahoney *et al.*, 1977). Over 65% of patients with Duchenne (and Becker) dystrophy have deletion mutations of one or more of the 65 unique exons that are distributed over the Duchenne locus at Xp21. If an affected family member is shown to have a deletion in this locus the fetus can be tested for this deletion by direct DNA analysis of chorionic villus tissue obtained at 10-weeks gestation. Karyotyping of this tissue enables fetal sex to be determined. RFLP analysis improves the accuracy of prenatal diagnosis (Cole *et al.*, 1988).

6.1.3 *Carrier detection*

Muscle biopsy has long been used as part of the investigation of a suspected carrier. Some carriers show hypertrophy of muscles and muscle biopsy may show muscle fibre hypertrophy in these cases. Other changes include increased central nucleation, increased variability in fibre size, fibre splitting and occasional basophilic fibres (Dubowitz and Brooke, 1973). However, these changes, when they occur, are usually slight; their absence does not exclude the carrier state. They are probably more common in young than in older carrier females. CK levels are raised in up to 70% of carriers (Griggs *et al.*, 1985). Immunohistochemical staining of muscle biopsies from putative carriers can be used to identify the carrier state in informative carriers. In some carriers a mosaic pattern of dystrophin reactivity is found on the surface membrane of muscle fibres in frozen sections. The sensitivity and specificity of this technique is uncertain (Bouilla *et al.*, 1988; Arahata *et al.*, 1989). Linkage analysis, and detection of intragenic DNA deletions in affected family members, are powerful diagnostic methods which greatly increase the accuracy of carrier detection in both Duchenne and Becker dystrophy (Hodgson and Bobrow, 1989).

6.2   Becker muscular dystrophy

This disorder is of later onset and slower progression than Duchenne dystrophy so that survival into adult life is usual and affected men may remain relatively mobile until the 4th decade. Becker muscular dystrophy is inherited as an X-linked disorder (Becker and Kiener, 1955), affecting the same dystrophin genetic system as Duchenne dystrophy, but it is less severe. In Becker muscular dystrophy dystrophin is present in an abnormal form, usually in a lower molecular weight configuration; in a few patients a larger molecule is produced and in some patients normal-sized dystrophin molecules are present in reduced amount (5–30% of normal) (Hoffman *et al.*, 1988; 1989). These abnormalities can be recognized by dystrophin immunoblot studies of freshly biopsied

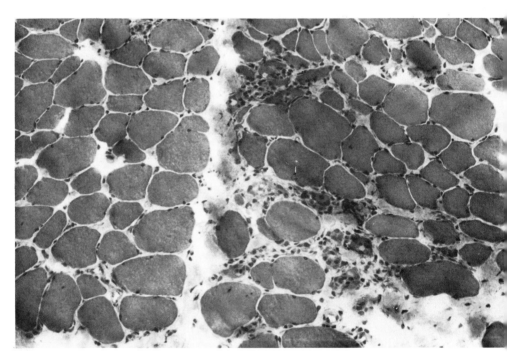

Fig. 6.8   Becker muscular dystrophy, × 180; HE. The abnormality in many respects resembles that of Duchenne muscular dystrophy, with marked regenerative fibre clusters.

muscle. This technique is probably the preferred method for diagnosis. The CK is raised to a similar degree to that found in Duchenne muscular dystrophy.

6.2.1   *Muscle pathology*

The muscle biopsy resembles that of Duchenne muscular dystrophy in some respects, particularly in the presence of rounded fibres, central nucleation, split fibres and endomysial fibrosis, but there are several points of difference. Hyaline fibres are relatively uncommon, fibre-type differentiation is not impaired, and clusters of small, angular NADH-dark fibres are often a feature (Bradley *et al.*, 1978). The latter may suggest a neurogenic process but the widespread dystrophic change is distinctive and diagnostic of the disorder (Fig. 6.8).

6.3   Other X-linked dystrophies

Several mild forms of X-linked muscular dystrophy have been described. Clinically, these cases resemble Becker's dystrophy, although they may begin even later, and follow a milder course. Only few such families have been described (Mabry *et al.*, 1965; Ringel *et al.*, 1977). The muscle biopsy shows features resembling Duchenne- and Becker-type muscular dystrophies in that hyaline fibres are present and there is variability in fibre size, with central nucleation and some increase in endomysial fibrous tissue. However, the histological abnormality is relatively less severe. A mild form of X-linked muscular dystrophy with a raised blood CK level and with acanthocytosis is associated with Kell blood group antigen (McLeod phenotype), and is also associated with the Xp21 locus (Swash *et al.*, 1983). An X-linked form of scapuloperoneal muscular dystrophy has also been reported; its histological features resemble those of limb-girdle muscular dystrophy.

6.4   Limb-girdle muscular dystrophy

The limb-girdle dystrophy syndrome (Walton and Nattrass, 1954) consists of a wide spectrum of progressive muscular disorders with a variable pattern of inheritance, although an autosomal recessive trait is common. Muscular weakness usually becomes apparent in the 2nd or 3rd decade and progresses slowly so that disability becomes severe only 20 years or more after the onset of the disorder. The CK level is raised, but not to the degree found in Duchenne dystrophy. Many cases formerly classified as limb-girdle muscular dystrophy have been found on reinvestigation, using modern enzyme histochemical muscle biopsy techniques, to have a neurogenic basis for their muscular weakness, usually spinal muscular atrophy of the Kugelberg–Welander type.

6.4.1   Muscle pathology

The muscle biopsy shows typical myopathic features (Fig. 6.9). In some biopsies muscle fibre hypertrophy is prominent, with muscle fibres up to 200 μm in transverse diameter. Central nucleation and fibre splitting may also be prominent. Various other morphological changes including whorled fibres (Fig. 6.10), sarcoplasmic masses, vacuolated fibres and peripheral accumulations of NADH-dark material may occur. Scattered necrotic and regenerating fibres are found but these are not prominent features of this slowly progressive disorder. Endomysial and interfascicular fibrosis and fat replacement occur in the advanced stages of the disorder (Fig. 6.11), when there has been extensive loss of muscle fibres. Small rounded atrophic fibres may persist in areas of fibrous tissue, amongst scattered or isolated hypertrophied fibres. Sparse

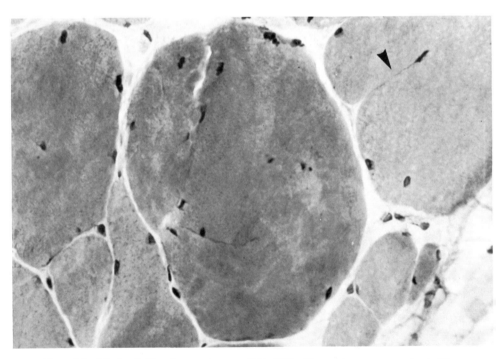

Fig. 6.9 Limb-girdle dystrophy, × 427; HE. There is very marked fibre hypertrophy. One fibre (arrow) is undergoing splitting – another shows an artefactual split induced during section processing.

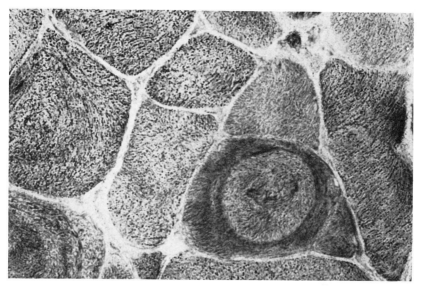

Fig. 6.10 Limb-girdle dystrophy, × 350; NADH. Fibre hypertrophy is prominent. A whorled fibre, in which abnormalities of myofilament orientation and distribution are accompanied by similar changes in mitochondrial distribution, is a very striking abnormality.

lymphocytic infiltration, often also containing macrophages, may be found in association with necrotic or regenerating fibres. Generally proximal leg muscles show more abnormality than proximal arm muscles and quadriceps biopsies are therefore more likely to show typical abnormalities than deltoid biopsies. Sometimes the vastus medialis is more atrophic than the lateral part of the quadriceps.

In some cases more specific histological abnormalities have been recognized. For example, the presence of extensively vacuolated Type 1 fibres, with dense accumulation of glycogen and acid phosphatase-positive material, is a feature associated with acid maltase deficiency (Type II glycogenosis), a disorder which may present in adult life as a slowly progressive myopathy resembling the syndrome of limb-girdle dystrophy (Engel, 1970; Hudgson *et al.*, 1968). Although there are variations in the pathological features of individual cases of limb-girdle dystrophy no specific features have been recognized and definitive subclassification of this syndrome has not yet been accomplished. The limb-girdle dystrophy syndrome represents a clinical syndrome that probably comprises a number of as yet unascertained genetic and metabolic muscular disorders.

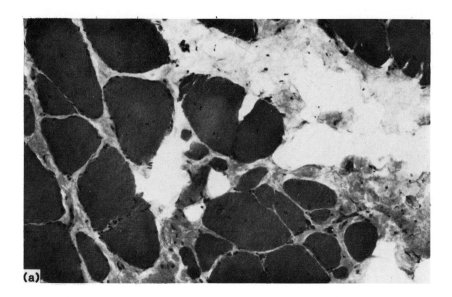

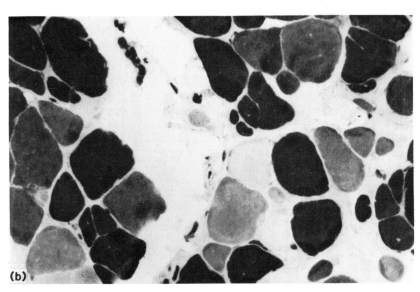

Fig. 6.11 Limb-girdle dystrophy. × 140 (a) HE. There is marked fibre hypertrophy, but also fibre atrophy, rounded fibres, fibre splitting, fibrosis, fat replacement, and increased central nucleation. (b) ATPase, pH 4.3. There is marked variation in fibre size, with increased numbers of Type 2C fibres (the fibres with an intermediate reaction between the dark Type 1 and pale Type 2A and Type 2B fibres). Fibre splitting is occurring in several fibres.

An important disorder to be considered in the differential diagnosis of limb-girdle muscular dystrophy is low-grade, or chronic polymyositis. This disorder can usually be readily differentiated by muscle biopsy, particularly by the presence of inflammatory cell infiltrates, when this occurs. Polymyositis is also characterized by active necrosis and re-generation, and by prominent architectural changes in individual fibres. Polymyositis, in addition, often shows a rather focal distribution of abnormality. Metabolic myopathy should be considered when there are ragged-red fibres, or when other inclusions are found in muscle fibres.

6.5   Facioscapulohumeral muscular dystrophy

This rare disorder is inherited as an autosomal dominant trait. Weakness usually involves face and shoulder-girdle musculature, particularly biceps brachii and periscapular muscles. Involvement of the leg muscles occurs later, particularly affecting anterior tibial muscles. Facial weakness may be a prominent presenting feature in childhood with little other abnormality until middle age but a severe childhood-onset form of the disease has also been described.

6.5.1   Muscle biopsy

In many patients the biopsy may be virtually normal, with occasional small round fibres as the only abnormal feature (Fig. 6.12). Since the shoulder girdle muscles are preferentially affected abnormalities are more prominent in upper than in lower limb muscles and biopsies should therefore always be taken from biceps brachii or deltoid muscles. Even in weak muscles abnormalities are not as striking as in other muscular dystrophies. Some fibres, especially Type 1 fibres, show whorled or moth-eaten changes (Dubowitz and Brooke, 1973) and small angular fibres, strongly reactive in oxidative enzyme reactions (e.g. NADH), are often found. The latter do not occur in groups as in neurogenic disorders. Hypertrophic fibres are also common but central nucleation and fibre splitting are infrequent and fibrosis is rare.

In some cases an inflammatory cell reaction may be a striking feature, and it may appear nodular (Munsat et al., 1972). In the more rapidly progressive cases this inflammatory change is sometimes associated with necrotic fibres but necrotic and regenerating fibres are uncommon in most cases of facioscapulohumeral dystrophy and the significance of this inflammatory cell reaction is unknown. Munsat et al. (1972) and Munsat and Bradley (1977) considered that some of these patients might be suffering from polymyositis, but there is no response to steroid treatment

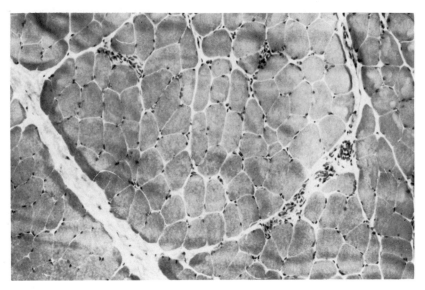

Fig. 6.12 Facioscapulohumeral dystrophy. × 140; HE. There are only mild abnormalities consisting of a few small fibres and increased perimysial and endomysial fibrous connective tissue. Nerve fibres are prominent. Fibre necrosis and other changes are not a feature.

in this form of muscular dystrophy. The differential diagnosis can be made by the family history, and by the presence of hypertrophied fibres, which are uncommon in polymyositis, even in the chronic phase.

Van Wijngaarden and Bethlem (1973) in a review of patients with weakness in a facioscapulohumeral distribution, mostly of sporadic occurrence, noted that a wide variety of neuromuscular disorders might be responsible, including polymyositis, myasthenia gravis, congenital myopathies and mitochondrial myopathies, in addition to facioscapulo-humeral dystrophy.

6.6   Distal myopathies

Distal myopathy was recognized as an autosomal dominant disorder in Sweden by Welander (1951); in this condition weakness begins in the hands and arms and later involves the feet. Type 1 fibre atrophy and central nucleation is followed by more marked myopathic features with vacuolar change as the disease progresses. Non-Swedish cases may be autosomal dominant or sporadic; the biopsy in these cases often shows prominent rimmed vacuoles of autophagic type with fibre necrosis and regeneration (Kratz and Brooke, 1979). In sporadic cases other abnormalities have been described, including focal granular degenerative change resembling a vacuolar appearance (Swash *et al.*, 1988).

6.7   Myotonic dystrophy

Myotonic dystrophy is a dominantly inherited disorder, with a genetic locus on the long arm of chromosome 19 near the apoprotein gene cluster, which shows marked variability in severity within individual pedigrees. The mutation rate for this disorder is low. Since mild forms of the disease are common, the diagnosis is often missed. On the other hand, the typical clinical features are well-known and in patients with the fully developed disorder muscle biopsy is usually not required for diagnosis. Furthermore, muscle biopsy is not useful in the diagnosis of patients in whom there is clinical uncertainty. Electromyography is far more useful, since it allows detection of the characteristic myotonia and provides evidence for a myopathy.

The most important clinical features are myotonia, weakness more marked in distal than in proximal muscles, causing weakness of the hands, and foot drop. The tendon reflexes are often absent. Systemic involvement is usual and includes cataract, endocrine disturbances, e.g. diabetes mellitus, testicular atrophy and infertility, dysphagia from involvement of the smooth muscle of the oesophagus, respiratory distress, and abnormalities of cardiac conduction including heart block. Mental abnormalities are frequent. Among affected adults men and women are equally affected, but the children of mothers with the disease may show a severe abnormality, with failure to thrive, respiratory distress, floppiness and weakness, marked facial weakness and mental retardation. The children of fathers with the disease are unlikely to develop this syndrome of *congenital myotonic dystrophy*.

6.7.1   Muscle biopsy

In the adult form of myotonic dystrophy the major abnormality is central nucleation (Fig. 6.13); frequently chains of central nuclei or multiple internal nuclei may be found (Figs 6.13 and 6.14). This is best seen in longitudinal sections. Very small fibres containing aggregations of dense nuclei are common and there is increased variability in fibre size (Fig. 6.15), with selective atrophy of Type 1 fibres, and hypertrophy of Type 2 fibres. Fibre splitting is sometimes prominent and ring fibres, in which displaced myofibrils appear to encircle the fibre beneath the plasma membrane in transverse sections, are an especially characteristic, but non-specific feature (Fig. 6.16). Sarcoplasmic masses, consisting of zones

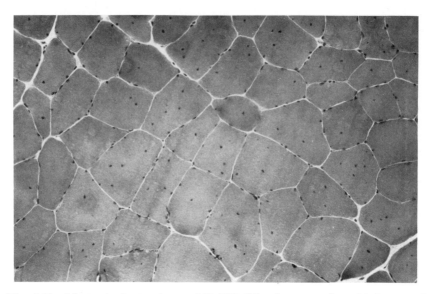

Fig. 6.13 Myotonic dystrophy. × 140; HE. Fibre hypertrophy with increased central nucleation are the main features (mean fibre diameter 81 μm; approximately 3 central nuclei per muscle fibre – the normal is < 0.04 central nuclei per muscle fibre).

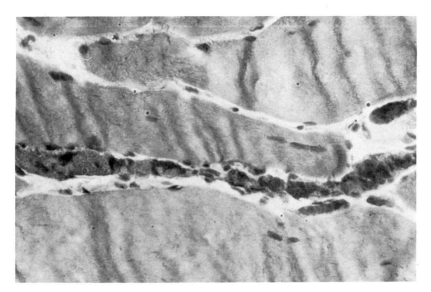

Fig. 6.14 Myotonic dystrophy. × 350; HE. This longitudinal section shows the tendency for internal nuclei to be arranged in chains (usually not a striking phenomenon), and the characteristic, slightly basophilic, tiny atrophic fibres, containing large, dark nuclei. The latter fibres resemble those found in chronic denervation atrophy. The wavy appearance is an artefact of section preparation.

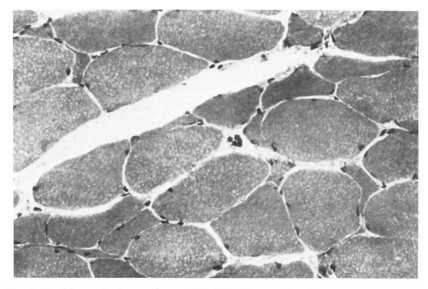

Fig. 6.15   Myotonic dystrophy. × 350; HE. The smaller fibres are more darkly stained (eosinophilic). These are atrophic Type 1 fibres. Central nucleation is not always a feature of the disease.

of clear or granular sarcoplasm, occur at the periphery of muscle fibres, both in adult- and childhood-onset cases.

The most characteristic abnormality in the muscle biopsy in myotonic dystrophy is found in the muscle spindles (Daniel and Strich, 1964). This abnormality is likely to be detected only in biopsies taken from distal muscles, e.g. flexor muscles of the forearm, since the disease affects distal muscles more than proximal muscles, and spindles are found in greater number in distal than in proximal muscles. The change consists of fragmentation of the intrafusal muscle fibres, so that there appears to be a marked increase in the number of intrafusal muscle fibres in affected spindles (Fig. 6.17). Thickening and fibrosis of the spindle capsule are also features of the abnormality. Normal spindles contain less than 14 intrafusal fibres but in myotonic dystrophy there may be as many as 100 separate tiny fragments in a single spindle in transverse section (Swash, 1972). Ultrastructural studies show a marked variation in the appearance of individual fibre fragments (Swash and Fox, 1975a; b), which is well demonstrated in serial sections. Not all the muscle spindles in a given muscle are abnormal, but the innervation of these abnormal spindles is disturbed, with marked proliferation of sensory and motor axons (Swash, 1972).

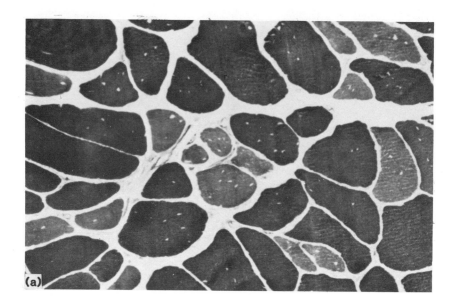

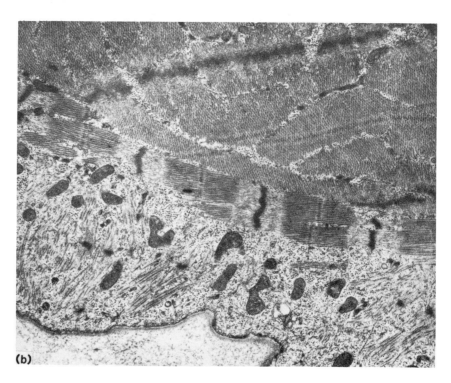

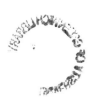

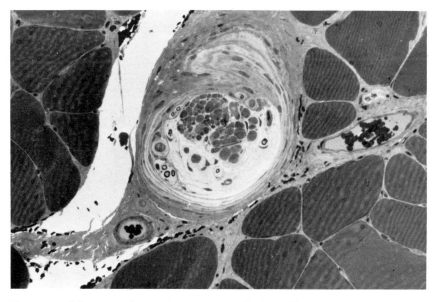

Fig. 6.17 Myotonic dystrophy. × 350; Toluidine blue, plastic section. The intrafusal muscle fibres are fragmented, either because of multiple splitting, or from abortive regenerative activity. The spindle capsule is thickened.

The motor innervation of extrafusal muscle fibres is also abnormal. There is expansion of the terminal arborization and prominent axonal branching leading to innervation of several adjacent muscle fibres by these branches (Coërs *et al.*, 1973).

In congenital myotonic dystrophy the biopsy is less abnormal. Central nucleation and fibre hypertrophy occur and sarcoplasmic masses may sometimes be prominent, but ring fibres are rarely a feature.

6.7.2 Other myotonic syndromes

There are two forms of myotonia congenita, a familial disorder characterized by myotonia without dystrophic features or signs of multisystem involvement. Muscle hypertrophy occurs in both the *dominantly inherited form* (Thomsen's disease) and in the *recessive form*

Fig. 6.16 Myotonic dystrophy. × 140; (a) ATPase, pH 9.5. Type 2 atrophy, with multiple central nucleation in fibres of both histochemical types, can be a distinctive feature of the disease. (b) Myotonic dystrophy. EM × 15 000. A peripheral myofibril is displaced into a 'ring' position, and there is a peripheral sarcoplasmic mass.

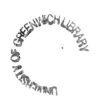

(Becker's variant) but in the latter, mild distal atrophy and weakness may develop in the course of the disease. *Paramyotonia congenita*, in which myotonia is markedly enhanced by cold, is also inherited as a dominant trait without systemic involvement.

The muscle biopsy in these conditions shows fibre hypertrophy with increased central nucleation, and there may be some scattered atrophic fibres (Fig. 6.18). Type 2B fibres may be absent both in the dominant and recessive forms (Crews *et al.*, 1976). Necrotic fibres may occur in the recessive form but are not a feature of autosomal dominant myotonia. Muscle spindles are normal in the recessive form (Swash and Schwartz, 1983).

6.8   Ocular myopathies and oculopharyngeal dystrophy

Ptosis and chronic progressive external ophthalmoplegia, due to muscular rather than cranial nerve or central nervous system disease,

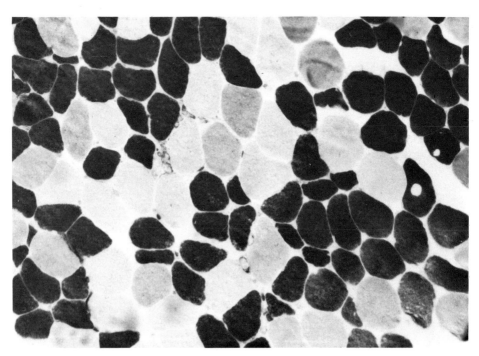

Fig. 6.18   Myotonia congenita. × 152; ATPase, pH 4.6. Scattered atrophic fibres (< 30 μm) without hypertrophic fibres. Two fibres are vacuolated, or show core formation.

may occur alone or in association with weakness of pharyngeal muscles. In many patients there is slight associated weakness of proximal muscles, especially of the upper limbs.

6.8.1 Muscle biopsy

Limb muscle biopsies in oculopharyngeal dystrophy show minor abnormalities including variability in fibre size with some hypertrophied fibres, scattered small angular fibres, darkly reactive in NADH preparations, some whorled or moth-eaten fibres but no necrotic or degenerating fibres. Ultrastructural studies have revealed filamentous inclusions in muscle fibre nuclei in this condition (Tomé and Fardeau, 1980).

In oculocraniosomatic syndrome systemic involvement, including cerebellar ataxia, deafness, retinitis pigmentosa, heart block and corticospinal signs, may occur. In this syndrome muscle biopsy may reveal ragged-red fibres, a feature suggesting mitochondrial myopathy (Chapter 8). Central core disease, and related syndromes may also cause mild proximal weakness with involvement of the external ocular muscles (Chapter 7).

References

Arahata, K., Ishihara, T., Kamakura, K. *et al.* (1989) Mosaic expression of dystrophin in symptomatic carriers of Duchenne's muscular dystrophy. *N. Engl. J. Med.*, **320**, 138–142.
Bell, C.D. and Conen, P.E. (1968) Histopathological changes in Duchenne muscular dystrophy. *J. Neurol. Sci.*, **7**, 529–544.
Becker, P.E. and Kiener, F. (1955) Eine neue X chromosale Muskel dystrophie. *Arch. Psychiat. Nervenkr.*, **193**, 427–448.
Bodensteiner, J.B. and Engel, A.G. (1978) Intracellular calcium accumulation in Duchenne dystrophy and other myopathies: a study of 567,000 muscle fibres in 114 biopsies. *Neurology*, **28**, 439–446.
Bouilla, E., Schmidt, B., Samitt, L.E. *et al.* (1988) Normal and dystrophin deficient muscle fibres in carriers of the gene for Duchenne muscular dystrophy. *Am. J. Pathol.*, **133**, 440–445.
Bradley, W.G., Jones, M.Z., Mussini, J.M. and Fawcett, P.R.W. (1978) Becker-type muscular dystrophy. *Muscle Nerve*, **1**, 111–132.
Carpenter, S. and Karpati, G. (1979) Duchenne muscular dystrophy: plasma membrane loss initiates muscle cell necrosis unless it is repaired. *Brain*, **102**, 147–161.
Coërs, C. and Tellerman-Toppet, N. (1977) Morphological changes of motor units in Duchenne's muscular dystrophy. *Arch. Neurol.*, **34**, 396–402.
Coërs, C., Tellerman-Toppet, N. and Gerard, J.-M. (1973) Terminal innervation ratio in neuromuscular disease: disorders of lower motor neuron, peripheral nerve and muscle. *Arch. Neurol.*, **29**, 215–222.
Cole, C.G., Walker, A., Coyne, A. *et al.* (1988) Prenatal testing for Duchenne and Becker muscular dystrophy. *Lancet*, **1**, 262–266.

128   Muscular dystrophies

Crews, J., Kaiser, K.K. and Brooke, M.H. (1976) Muscle pathology of myotonia congenita. *J. Neurol. Sci.*, **28**, 449–457.

Cullen, M.J. and Fulthorpe, J.J. (1975) Stages in fibre breakdown in Duchenne muscular dystrophy. An electromicroscopic study. *J. Neurol. Sci.*, **24**, 179–200.

Daniel, P.M. and Strich, S.J. (1964) Abnormalities in the muscle spindles in dystrophia myotonica. *Neurology*, **14**, 310–316.

Dubowitz, V. and Brooke, M.H. (1973) *Muscle Biopsy – A Modern Approach*, W.B. Saunders, London.

Emery, A.E.H. and Burt, D.E. (1980) Intracellular calcium and pathogenesis and antenatal diagnosis of Duchenne muscular dystrophy. *Br. Med. J.*, **280**, 355–357.

Engel, A.G. (1970) Acid maltase deficiency in adults. *Brain*, **93**, 599–606.

Engel, W.K. (1977) Integrative histochemical approach to the defect in muscular dystrophy. In *Pathogenesis of Human Muscular Dystrophies* (ed. L.P. Rowland), Excerpta Medica, Amsterdam, pp. 277–309.

Griggs, R.C., Mendell, J.R., Brooke, M.H. *et al.* (1985) Clinical investigation in Duchenne muscular dystrophy V. Use of creatine kinase and pyruvate kinase in carrier detection. *Muscle Nerve*, **8**, 60–67.

Harper, P.S. (1982) Carrier detection in Duchenne muscular dystrophy: a critical assessment. In *Disorders of the Motor Unit* (ed. D.L. Schotland), Wiley Medical, New York, ch. 63, pp. 821–846.

Hodgson, S.V. and Bobrow, M. (1989) Carrier detection and prenatal diagnosis in Duchenne and Becker muscular dystrophy. *Br. Med. Bull.*, **45**, 719–744.

Hoffman, E.P., Fischbeck, K.H., Brown, R.H. *et al.* (1988) Characterisation of dystrophin in muscle biopsy specimens from patients with Duchenne's or Becker's muscular dystrophy. *N. Engl. J. Med.*, **318**, 1363–1368.

Hoffman, E.P., Kunkel, L.M., Angelini, C. *et al.* (1989) Improved diagnosis of Becker muscular dystrophy by dystrophin testing. *Neurology*, **39**, 1011–1017.

Hudgson, P., Gardner-Medwin, D., Worsfold, M. *et al.* (1968) Adult myopathy from glycogen storage disease due to acid maltase deficiency. *Brain*, **91**, 435–462.

Kratz, R. and Brooke, M.H. (1979) Distal myopathy. In *Diseases of Muscle (Handbook of Clinical Neurology)* (eds P.J. Vinken, G.W. Bruyn and S.J. Ringel), North Holland, Amsterdam, vol. **40**, pp. 471–483.

Kunkel, L.M. and Hoffman, E.P. (1989) Duchenne/Becker muscular dystrophy. *Br. Med. Bull.*, **45**, 630–643.

Mabry, C.C., Rockel, I.E., Morwick, R.L. and Robertson, D. (1965) X-linked pseudo hypertrophic muscular dystrophy with a late onset and slow progression. *N. Engl. J. Med.*, **273**, 1062–1070.

Mahoney, M.J., Haseltine, F.P. and Hobbins, J.C. (1977) Prenatal diagnosis of Duchenne muscular dystrophy. *N. Engl. J. Med.*, **297**, 968–973.

Mokri, B. and Engel, A.G. (1975) Duchenne dystrophy: electron microscopic findings pointing to a basic or early abnormality in the plasma membrane of the muscle fibre. *Neurology*, **25**, 1111–1120.

Munsat, T.L. and Bradley, W.G. (1977) Serum creatine phosphokinase levels and prednisone-treated muscle weakness. *Neurology*, **27**, 96–97.

Munsat, T.L., Piper, O., Canulla, P. and Mednik, J. (1972) Inflammatory myopathy with facio-scapulo-humeral distribution. *Neurology*, **22**, 335–347.

Neerunjun, S.J.S. and Dubowitz, V. (1977) Concomitance of basophilia, ribonucleic acid and acid phosphatase activity in regenerating muscle fibres. *J. Neurol. Sci.*, **33**, 95–109.

Ringel, S.P., Carroll, J.E. and Schold, S.C. (1977) The spectrum of mild X-linked recessive muscular dystrophy. *Arch. Neurol.*, **34**, 408–416.

Swash, M. (1972) The morphology and innervation of the muscle spindle in dystrophic myotonica. *Brain*, **95**, 357–368.

Swash, M. and Fox, K.P. (1975a) Abnormal intrafusal muscle fibres in myotonic dystrophy: a study using serial sections. *J. Neurol. Neurosurg. Psychiatry*, **38**, 91–99.

Swash, M. and Fox, K.P. (1975b) The fine structure of the spindle abnormality in myotonic dystrophy. *Neuropathol. Appl. Neurobiol.*, **1**, 171–187.

Swash, M. and Fox, K.P. (1976) The pathology of the muscle spindle in Duchenne muscular dystrophy. *J. Neurol. Sci.*, **29**, 17–32.

Swash, M. and Schwartz, M.S. (1983) Normal muscle spindle morphology in myotonia congenita. *Clin. Neuropathol.*, **2**, 75–78.

Swash, M., Schwartz, M.S., Carter, N.D. *et al.* (1983) Benign X-linked myopathy with acanthocytes (McLeod syndrome) – its relationship to X-linked muscular dystrophy. *Brain*, **106**, 717–734.

Swash, M., Schwartz, M.S., Thompson, A. *et al.* (1988) Distal myopathy with focal granular degenerative change in vacuolated Type 2 fibres. *Clin. Neuropathol.*, **7**, 249–253.

Tomé, F. and Fardeau, M. (1980) Nuclear inclusions in oculopharyngeal dystrophy. *Acta Neuropathol. (Berlin)*, **49**, 85–87.

van Wijngaarden, G.K. and Bethlem, J. (1973) The facio-scapulo-humeral syndrome. In *Clinical Studies in Myology* (ed. B.A. Kakulas), Excerpta Medica, Amsterdam, pp. 498–501.

Walton, J.N. (1973) Progressive muscular dystrophy: structural alteration in various stages and in carriers of muscular dystrophy. In *The Striated Muscle* (ed. C.M. Pearson), Williams and Wilkins, Baltimore, pp. 263–291.

Walton, J.N. and Gardner-Medwin, D. (1981) Progressive muscular dystrophy and the myotonic disorders. In *Disorders of Voluntary Muscle*, 4th edn (ed. J.N. Walton), Churchill Livingstone, Edinburgh, pp. 481–524.

Walton, J.N. and Nattrass, F.T. (1954) On the classification, natural history and treatment of the myopathies. *Brain*, **77**, 169–231.

Welander, L. (1951) Myopathia distalis tarda hereditaria. *Acta Med. Scand.*, Suppl. **265**, 1–124.

Zubrzycka-Gaarn, E.E., Bulman, D.E., Karpati, G. *et al.* (1988) The Duchenne muscular dystrophy gene product is localised in the sarcolemma of human skeletal muscle fibres. *Nature*, **333**, 466–469.

7 'Benign' myopathies of childhood

The term 'benign myopathies of childhood' is used to describe a group of disorders sometimes referred to as congenital myopathies, although in some instances they may not cause symptoms until later in childhood or even until adult life. These disorders usually have a genetic basis, although this may not be apparent. In most patients weakness is mild or moderate, and marked wasting is unusual. These disorders are usually only slowly progressive and, in some, improvement may occur with increasing maturity (Dubowitz, 1978; 1980).

Many of the children present in infancy with the 'floppy infant

Table 7.1 Causes of floppy infant syndrome

Central nervous system disease
    Cerebral palsy
    Mental retardation
    Cerebellar disease
    Spinal cord injury

Neurogenic disorders
    Type 1 spinal atrophy (Werdnig–Hoffman)
    Poliomyelitis
    Peripheral neuropathy

Infantile myasthenia gravis

Myopathies
    Congenital muscular dystrophy
    Myopathies with structural changes in the muscle biopsy (see Table 7.2)
    Metabolic myopathies of childhood (see Chapter 8)
    Myotonic dystrophy

Others (usually without weakness)
    Benign congenital hypotonia
    Ehlers–Danlos and related syndromes
    Prader–Willi syndrome
    Reversible metabolic disorders, e.g. hypoglycaemia
    Hypothyroidism and other endocrine disorders

Table 7.2 'Benign' myopathies of childhood (childhood-onset myopathies with slow progression and structural changes in the muscle biopsy)

Nemaline myopathy
Central core and multicore (minicore) disease
Centronuclear (myotubular) myopathy
Congenital fibre-type disproportion
Myopathy with tubular aggregates
Failure of fibre-type differentiation

Others
  Myopathy with fingerprint inclusions
  Zebra body myopathy
  Minimal-change myopathy
  Congenital muscular dystrophy

syndrome'. This syndrome consists of reduced resistance of joints to passive movement and increased range of joint movement. Affected infants usually show reduced spontaneous movements and older children have delayed motor milestones. The floppy infant syndrome has many causes (Table 7.1). These are classified according to their underlying cause, e.g. as metabolic myopathies, etc., leaving a group of ill-understood, relatively benign myopathies of childhood that are characterized principally by the changes found in the muscle biopsy (Table 7.2). In some cases no underlying cause can be found and, with increasing maturity, the hypotonia resolves (Dubowitz, 1980).

Hypotonia occurring in children of normal intelligence, with retained tendon reflexes and normal active movements of the limbs, is unlikely to have a serious or progressive underlying cause. If improvement occurs in a few months and the CK is normal, no further investigation is required. Lundberg (1979) found that only 4% of a group of children had an underlying neuromuscular disorder. In a series of infants with hypotonia, associated with other features of neurological disorder, Paine (1963) found that 73% had central nervous system disease, 16% were categorized as benign congenital myopathy and 3% had a myopathy or spinal muscular atrophy, respectively. Myopathies of infancy and childhood are thus uncommon disorders.

7.1 Nemaline myopathy

This is probably the commonest of the congenital myopathies presenting in childhood. The disease may present in infancy or in childhood; the disorder varies greatly in severity from case to case. Martinez and Lake (1987) recognized three major clinical syndromes:

1. A severe neonatal syndrome, with autosomal recessive inheritance and a fatal outcome before the age of 2 years. Respiratory problems, absent tendon reflexes and dysmorphic features including kyphoscoliosis and pes cavus are evident.
2. A mild form with autosomal dominant inheritance. This syndrome is the commonest form of nemaline myopathy and although slowly progressive the outcome is favourable.
3. Adult-onset nemaline myopathy, usually mild and sporadic, but occasionally accompanied by fatal cardiomyopathy.

7.1.1   Muscle biopsy

The pathology is similar in all clinical forms of the disease, regardless of the rate of progression of weakness. The cardinal feature is the presence of rod-like inclusions (Fig. 7.1), which appear red in the Gomori trichrome preparation, faintly basophilic in HE stains, and blue in PTAH preparations. In HE stains they are best seen by phase microscopy (Hudgson *et al.*, 1967); their optical density resembles that of the Z-discs. The rod bodies are usually mainly subsarcolemmal and paranuclear in location. They vary in length from 1 to 5 μm and in diameter from 0.2 to

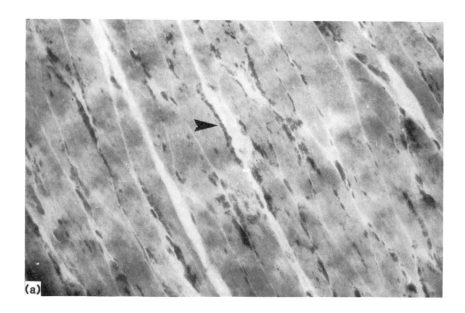

(a)

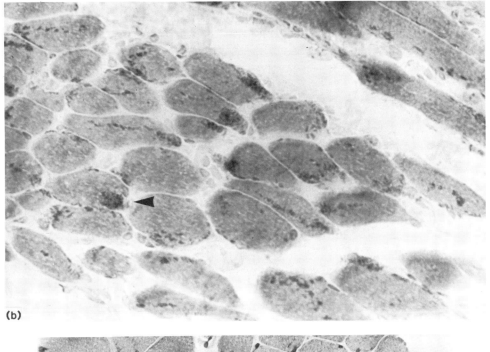

(b)

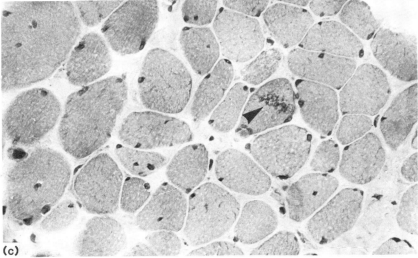

(c)

Fig. 7.1 (a) Nemaline myopathy. × 560; Gomori trichrome, longitudinal section. Child aged 2 years. The characteristic rod bodies are located in the subsarcolemmal region. They are arranged in clumps; note their small size, and the absence of other abnormality in the fibres. (b) Transverse section of same case as (a). × 617. (c) Rod bodies. × 350; Gomori trichrome. In this adult muscle the rod bodies were a non-specific and less prominent abnormality than in the typical infantile-onset cases.

2.0 μm (Bethlem, 1980). They can been seen in both Type 1 and Type 2 fibres and even in the intrafusal muscle fibres of the muscle spindles. In enzyme histochemical preparations they are non-reactive, appearing as pale areas. In most cases the presence of rod bodies is the only abnormality in the muscle biopsy, but in some cases scattered small fibres may be seen with increased central nucleation and there may be a predominance of Type 1 and Type 2C fibres. Rod bodies may coexist with cores (Afifi *et al.*, 1965) and with failure of fibre-type differentiation (Nienhuis *et al.*, 1967). Generally the numbers of rods found in muscle fibres increases as the disease progresses.

Ultrastructural studies (Fig. 7.2) show the rods to be rectangular and electron-dense. When situated in the myofibrils of a fibre they usually occupy a single sarcomere and seem to originate from the Z-bands of affected sarcomeres, but when found at the periphery of a fibre they lie in various orientations in granular cytoplasm without attachment to myofilaments. Their protein composition is uncertain but they react in histochemical preparations for tyrosine and are thought to consist of tropomyosin or actinin.

Rod bodies are a non-specific feature of degenerative change in myofibrils, and are seen in a few scattered fibres in a number of different disorders including many other myopathies and neurogenic disorders (Swash and Schwartz, 1988), in schizophrenics, in Parkinson's disease and in HIV infection (Dalakas *et al.*, 1987). In these disorders rod bodies are usually found in myofilaments and not in a subsarcolemmal location. They are also found in normal external ocular muscles, at the myotendinous junction in normal skeletal muscle, and in tenotomized muscle in the cat (Karpati *et al.*, 1972).

7.2   Central core disease

Central cores, multicores (minicores) and focal loss of cross-striations are related abnormalities which are difficult to classify separately since they may all occur in the same biopsy (Bethlem *et al.*, 1978; Swash and Schwartz, 1981). However, these abnormalities are usually regarded as pathognomonic of separate entities because each of these pathological features may occur alone, and because the clinical features, especially the occurrence of associated ophthalmoplegia in cases with focal loss of cross-striations, vary from case to case.

Central core disease was the first of the benign myopathies of childhood to be recognized. The major features consist of hypotonia, delay in achieving motor milestones and mild, non-progressive weakness (Shy and Magee, 1956) sometimes associated with skeletal abnormalities. Central core disease is usually a dominantly inherited disorder.

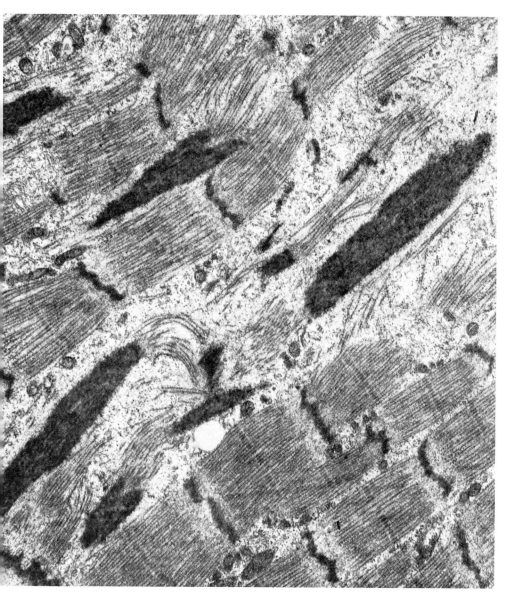

Fig. 7.2   Rod bodies. EM, × 21 000. The rod bodies are seen as granular electron-dense bodies with sharp borders, arising from Z-band material. In conditions other than nemaline myopathy, rod bodies often occur in association with zones of myofibrillar degeneration.

Susceptibility to malignant hyperthermia was recognized in 11 of 13 cases by Schuaib *et al.* (1987); all cases should be screened for this problem. *Multicore disease* usually presents in infancy. Contractures may develop, and cardiorespiratory complications may develop (Swash and Schwartz, 1981).

7.2.1 Muscle biopsy

In central core disease there is an abnormal central or somewhat eccentric zone within the transverse area of affected fibres. This zone shows reduced or absent oxidative enzyme activity, e.g. NADH (Fig. 7.3), and reduced reactivity in PAS preparations. In Gomori preparations this abnormal zone stains bluish but in HE the core region usually appears normal although it can be recognized with phase-contrast microscopy. Most cores occur in Type 1 fibres and there is often Type 1 predominance, and increased numbers of Type 2C fibres. In ATPase preparations (pH 4.3) the core regions may be reactive or unreactive. This difference

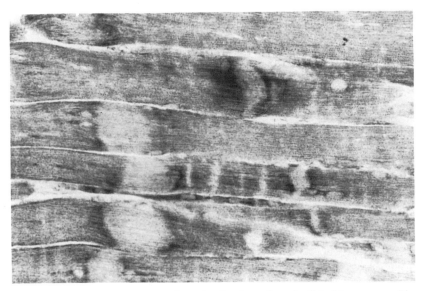

Fig. 7.3 Cores. × 560; NADH, Longitudinal section. In this biopsy core-like zones of non-reactivity are present. These contain degenerate myofibrils, and mitochondria are absent. In central core disease this abnormality (unstructured cores) extends through long segments of affected fibres, but in this case the abnormality is discrete. The latter is more typical of multicore disease. The slit-like zones of unreactivity are termed 'focal loss of cross-striations'.

has led to subdivision of the core abnormality into structured and unstructured types (Neville, 1978).

In structured cores the core region shows a normal or increased reaction with ATPase; and with the electron microscope this zone shows myofilaments slightly more contracted than in the surrounding normal area of the fibre. The Z-bands are irregular, widened or smeared, and mitochondria are absent.

In unstructured cores there is loss of the normal myofibrillar pattern, and of mitochondria, so that the regular striated appearance is lost and the ATPase reaction is negative. Unstructured cores resemble the early stage of target fibre formation (Fig. 7.4) and there is confusion in the nomenclature of these abnormalities (Schmitt and Volk, 1975; Swash and Schwartz, 1981; 1988).

Cores are usually said to extend through the length of affected fibres without interruption, but most longitudinal sections do not extend more than a few hundred micrometres at the most, and this is therefore a difficult point of which to be certain. By contrast, *multi(mini)cores* occur at multiple zones in the transverse area of affected fibres, usually Type 1 fibres, and extend only a short longitudinal distance. The edges of the

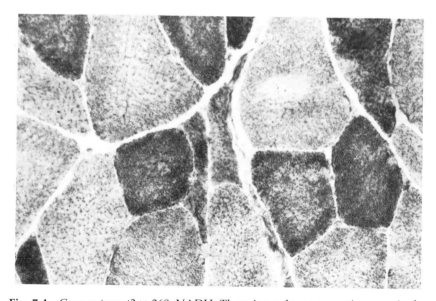

Fig. 7.4   Core or target? × 360; NADH. There is a pale, non-reactive zone in the pale Type 2 fibre at the top of the illustration which resembles a core. However, there is also a small cluster of NADH-dark, pointed, atrophic denervated fibres, suggesting denervation and thus implying that the 'core' is really a target (see text). A nearby dark Type 1 fibre shows a small central target-like abnormality.

lesions are sharply circumscribed. Central nucleation is more frequent in biopsies showing multicores than in central core disease itself. *Focal loss of cross-striations* (van Wijngaarden *et al.*, 1977) is a less common abnormality (Fig. 7.5), consisting of a linear transverse lucency in NADH preparations, resembling unstructured cores, but extending only a few sarcomeres in the length of the fibre (Fig. 7.6) (Swash and Schwartz, 1981). Sarcolemmal nuclei are often located close to zones of focal loss of cross-striations.

7.3 Centronuclear (myotubular) myopathy

In the severe neonatal form of this disorder, cardiopulmonary problems together with facial and bulbar weakness often lead to death in the first two years of life. This neonatal form is X-linked and has also been termed myotubular myopathy. External ophthalmoplegia may be a feature of these cases. Less severe forms of the disease, presenting in childhood or in adult life, may occur.

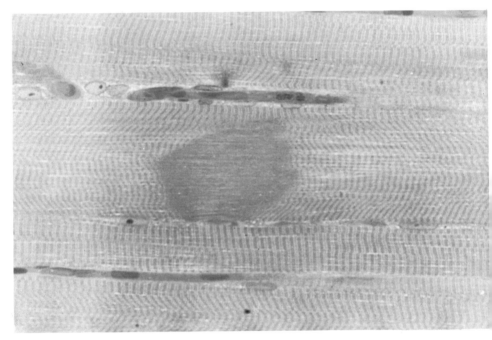

Fig. 7.5 Focal loss of cross-striations. × 532; Toluidine blue. The focal zone of loss of cross-striations is clearly evident in this semithin plastic-embedded section.

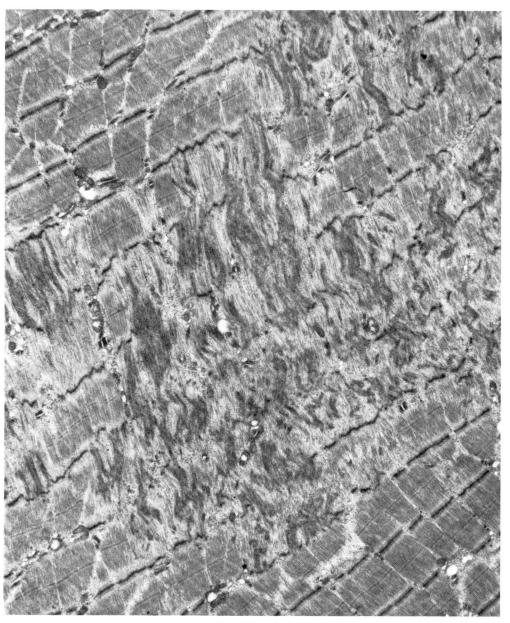

Fig. 7.6 Multicore disease. EM, × 8400. This unstructured core consists of a zone of disrupted myofilamentous and tubular material, lacking mitochondria. There is a relatively sudden transition to normal muscle at the edges of the lesion.

7.3.1   Muscle biopsy

The main abnormality is the presence of central nuclei in zones of affected fibres devoid of ATPase reactivity (Fig. 7.7). This central zone contains aggregates of mitochondria but few myofibrils and so lacks oxidative enzymatic activity, although it may contain glycogen and autophagic vacuoles. Type 1 fibres are affected more severely than Type 2 fibres. These fibres resemble fetal myotubes (Spiro *et al.*, 1966) but not all fibres show this perinuclear, clear zone.

7.4   Congenital fibre-type disproportion

This disorder presents with hypotonia, weakness and respiratory difficulties. Contractures and congenital dislocation of the hip are features of the disease (Cavanagh *et al.*, 1979). Inheritance may be dominant or recessive.

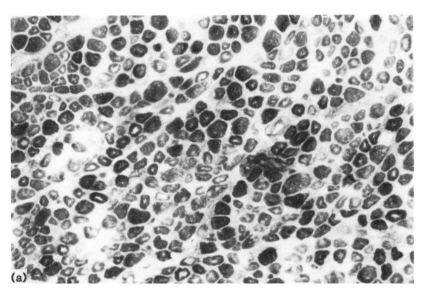

(a)

Fig. 7.7   (a) Centronuclear (myotubular) myopathy. × 350; ATPase, pH 4.3. Many of the fibres contain a central zone of non-reactivity, corresponding to the nucleus, and a perinuclear zone of absence of myofibrils. Note the small-sized muscle fibres characteristic of biopsies at this age (1 year). (b) HE and (c) ATPase, pH 9.5, × 427. Normal fetal myotubes. Abortion at 2 months gestation. In the limb the developing muscles are represented by clusters of normal myotubes. Their tubular form is seen in the ATPase preparation (c) and their central nuclei in the longitudinal HE stain (b). This stage of development is followed by maturation so that at birth myotubes are not normally present.

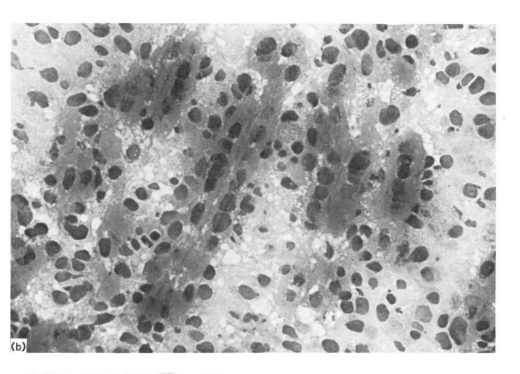
(b)

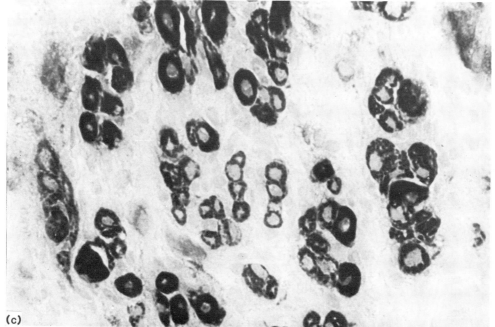
(c)

7.4.1 Muscle biopsy

In this disorder there is disproportion in the diameters of Type 1 and Type 2 fibres (Brooke, 1973). This disparity is due to hypertrophy of Type 2 fibres, especially Type 2B fibres, the Type 1 fibres being of normal size (Fig. 7.8). In order to establish the diagnosis the mean diameter of Type 1 fibres should be at least 12% less than that of the Type 2 fibres (Brooke, 1973). Associated abnormalities, including increased central nucleation, moth-eaten fibres and rod bodies, may also occur.

The disorder must be differentiated from Type 1 atrophy found in myotonic dystrophy and myotubular myopathy. The histological features may also sometimes resemble those found in the early stages of Werdnig–Hoffmann disease (Type 1 spinal muscular atrophy) but in the latter, fibre-type grouping is usually a feature and the large fibres in the latter condition may be undifferentiated. The finding of fibre-type disproportion may represent a non-specific pathological change, resulting from one of several different disorders, rather than a specific disease entity.

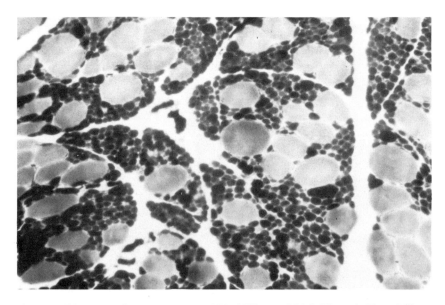

Fig. 7.8 Fibre-type disproportion. × 350; ATPase, pH 4.3. The pale Type 2 fibres are large and rounded. There is Type 1 fibre predominance but the Type 1 fibres are of a uniformly small size.

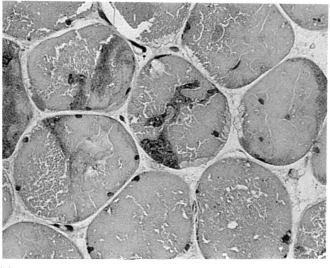

(b)

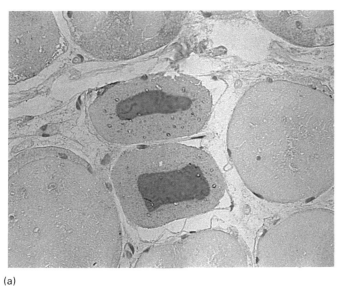

(a)

Fig. 7.9 Myopathy with tubular aggregates. (a) HE. × 360. There are accumulations of basophilic granular material that are clearly demarcated from the sarcoplasm of the affected fibres. This material is red-staining in Gomori, positive in NADH and negative in ATPase preparations. (b) Heat-shock protein (HSP 72) immunoperoxidase reaction. × 560. The HSP 72 is bound diffusely to the abnormal tubular matrix, indicating a role for this non-lysosomal protein degradation system in formation or lysis of these abnormal tubular aggregations.

7.5 Myopathy with tubular aggregates

Tubular aggregates are a rare phenomenon found most abundantly in Type 2 fibres in patients with pain and cramps on exertion (Morgan-Hughes *et al.*, 1970). A few cases of mild weakness with hypotonia in infancy have also been described in which tubular aggregates, usually restricted to Type 2B fibres but occasionally also found in Type 1 fibres (Dobkin and Verity, 1978), were the only abnormality. Tubular aggregates have also been reported in a slowly progressive limb-girdle myopathy syndrome. Tubular aggregates (Fig. 7.9) consist of clusters of closely packed tubules (Fig. 7.10), probably derived from the sarcoplasmic reticulum, which stain bright red in Gomori stains, are basophilic in HE, and which react positively in NADH preparations but negatively in SDH and in ATPase preparations. They express heat-shock proteins. Tubular abnormalities of less uniform structure, consisting of dilatation of the sarcoplasmic reticulum, or stacked tubules of varying size, occur in periodic paralysis, in myotonia congenita and in some patients with a congenital myasthenic syndrome (see Martin *et al.*, 1990).

7.6 Failure of fibre-type differentiation

In this rare disorder the muscle fibres fail to differentiate into fibre types in the ATPase preparations. Sometimes myopathic features may be present, for example, fat 'replacement' may be a feature.

7.7 Other benign myopathies of childhood

A number of other, extremely rare disorders without specific clinical features are recognized by their histological or ultrastructural appearances, for example, subsarcolemmal fingerprint inclusions (Engel *et al.*, 1972), zebra body myopathy (Lake and Wilson, 1975), etc. (see Mastaglia and Hudgson, 1981, for review). *Minimal change myopathy* is a term used to describe patients with weakness and reduced tone in whom the muscle biopsy is either normal or shows only minor abnormalities (Dubowitz, 1978). In some of these cases repeat biopsy reveals more distinct pathological features.

7.8 Congenital muscular dystrophy

This term is used to describe children in whom a non-progressive congenital myopathy with severe weakness, often associated with arthrogryposis, is accompanied by histological appearances in the muscle biopsy typical of muscular dystrophy. There may be severe abnormality

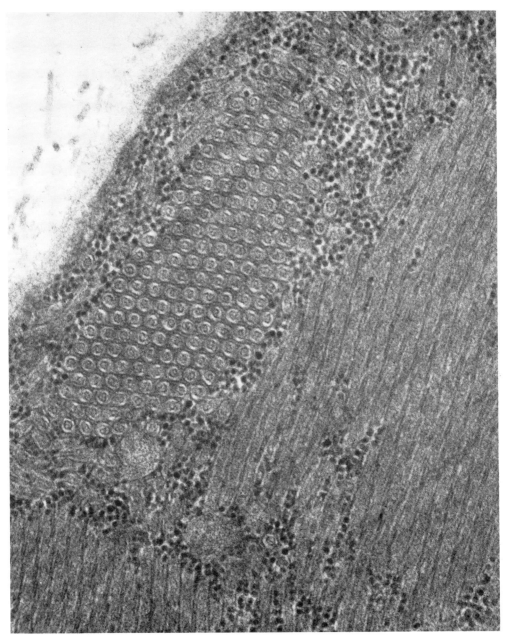

Fig. 7.10 Tubular aggregates. EM, × 70 200. Affected fibres show a peripheral, bright red, inclusion in the Gomori preparation consisting of stacked tubules derived from the sarcoplasmic reticulum. This abnormality is a non-specific finding. In this EM preparation the stacked tubular structure of this inclusion can be seen.

in the muscle biopsy, consisting of fibrosis and fat replacement, with marked variability in fibre size, although usually without active fibre necrosis and regeneration. The blood CK level, unlike that found in Duchenne muscular dystrophy, is normal or only slightly raised (Donner et al., 1975). In other cases only minimal pathological change may be found (Dubowitz, 1978).

References

Afifi, A.K., Smith, T.W. and Zellweger, H. (1965) Congenital non-progressive myopathy: central core and nemaline myopathy in one family. Neurology, 15, 371–381.

Bethlem, J. (1980) Myopathies, 2nd edn, Elsevier, Amsterdam.

Bethlem, J., Arts, W.F. and Dingemans, K.P. (1978) Common origin of rods, cores, miniature cores and focal loss of cross-striations. Arch. Neurol., 35, 555–566.

Brooke, M.H. (1973) Congenital fibre type disproportion. In Clinical Studies in Myology (ed. B.A. Kakulas), Excerpta Medica, Amsterdam, pp. 147–159.

Cavanagh, N.P.C., Lake, B.D. and McMeniman, P. (1979) Congenital fibre type disproportion myopathy: a histological diagnosis with an uncertain clinical outlook. Arch. Dis. Child., 54, 735–743.

Dalakas, M.C., Pezeshkpour, G.H. and Flaherty, M. (1987) Progressive nemaline (rod) myopathy associated with HIV infection. N. Engl. J. Med., 317, 1602–1603.

Dobkin, B.H. and Verity, M.A. (1978) Familial neuromuscular disease with Type 1 fibre hypoplasia, tubular aggregates, cardiomyopathy and myasthenic features. Neurology, 28, 1135–1140.

Donner, M., Rapola, J. and Somer, H. (1975) Congenital muscular dystrophy: a clinico-pathological and follow-up study of 15 patients. Neuropëdiatrie, 6, 239–258.

Dubowitz, V. (1978) Muscle Disorders in Childhood, W.B. Saunders, London.

Dubowitz, V. (1980) The Floppy Infant Syndrome, 2nd edn, Heinemann, London.

Engel, A.G., Angelini, C. and Gomez, M.R. (1972) Finger print body myopathy. Mayo Clin. Proc., 47, 377–388.

Hudgson, P., Gardner-Medwin, D., Fulthorpe, J.L. and Walton, J.N. (1967) Nemaline myopathy. Neurology, 17, 1125–1142.

Karpati, G., Carpenter, S. and Eisen, A.A. (1972) Experimental core-like lesions and nemaline rods. Arch. Neurol., 27, 237–251.

Lake, B.D. and Wilson, T. (1975) Zebra body myopathy: clinical, histochemical and ultrastructural studies. J. Neurol. Sci., 24, 437–446.

Lundberg, A. (1979) Dissociated motor development; developmental patterns, clinical characteristics; causal factors and outcome with special reference to late-walking children. Neuropëdiatrie, 10, 161–182.

Martin, J.E., Mather, K., Swash, M. and Gray, A. (1990) Expression of heat-shock protein epitopes in tubular aggregates. Muscle Nerve (in press).

Martinez, B.A. and Lake, B.D. (1987) Childhood nemaline myopathy: a review of clinical presentation in relation to prognosis. Dev. Med. Child. Neurol., 29, 815–820.

Mastaglia, F.L. and Hudgson, P. (1981) Ultrastructural studies of diseased muscle. In Disorders of Voluntary Muscle, 4th edn (ed. J.N. Walton), Churchill Livingstone, Edinburgh, pp. 296–356.

Morgan-Hughes, J.A., Mair, W.G.P. and Lascelles, P.T. (1970) A disorder of skeletal muscle associated with tubular aggregates. *Brain*, **93**, 873–880.

Neville, H.E. (1978) Ultrastructural changes in diseases of human skeletal muscle. In *Handbook of Clinical Neurology*, Vol. 40 (eds P.J. Vinken and G.W. Bruyn), North Holland, Amsterdam, pp. 63–124.

Nienhuis, A.W., Coleman, F.R., Brown, J.J. *et al.* (1967) Nemaline myopathy: a histopathologic and biochemical study. *Am. J. Clin. Pathol.*, **48**, 1–13.

Paine, R.S. (1963) The future of the floppy infant, a follow up study of 133 patients. *Dev. Med. Child Neurol.*, **5**, 115–124.

Schmitt, H.P. and Volk, B. (1975) The relationship between target, targetoid and targetoid-core fibres in severe neurogenic muscular atrophy. *J. Neurol.*, **210**, 167–181.

Schuaib, A., Passuke, R.T. and Brownell, K.W. (1987) Central core disease; clinical features in 13 patients. *Medicine*, **66**, 389–396.

Shy, G.M. and Magee, K.R. (1956) A new congenital non-progressive myopathy. *Brain*, **79**, 610–621.

Spiro, A.J., Shy, G.M. and Gonatas, N.K. (1966) Myotubular myopathy. *Arch. Neurol.*, **14**, 1–14.

Swash, M. and Schwartz, M.S. (1981) Familial multicore disease with focal loss of cross striations and ophthalmoplegia. *J. Neurol. Sci.*, **52**, 1–10.

Swash, M. and Schwartz, M.S. (1988) *Neuromuscular Diseases, A Practical Approach to Diagnosis and Management*, 2nd edn, Springer-Verlag, Berlin.

van Wijngaarden, G.K., Bethlem, J., Dingemans, K.P. *et al.* (1977) Familial focal loss of cross-striations. *J. Neurol.*, **216**, 163–172.

8 Metabolic, endocrine and drug-induced myopathies

The metabolic, endocrine and drug-induced myopathies are discussed in this chapter as a related group of disorders because, in a general sense, they share a common pathogenetic mechanism. The metabolic myopathies result from a biochemical defect in muscle metabolism itself, the endocrine myopathies from an abnormal hormonal environment, probably affecting muscle metabolism, and the drug-induced myopathies from a direct toxic effect of the drug on muscle metabolism. In some drug-induced myopathies, e.g. malignant hyperpyrexia myopathy, the drug effect is manifest only in susceptible individuals.

8.1 Metabolic myopathies

The clinical features of this group of disorders vary considerably. Their severity ranges from benign muscle cramps to a presentation resembling the limb-girdle syndrome with marked muscular atrophy. In some instances acute episodes of myoglobinuria may occur, and in others, e.g. the periodic paralyses, attacks of severe flaccid weakness with rapid recovery are a feature. Exercise may precipitate symptoms in many of these metabolic disorders. The main types of metabolic myopathy are shown in Table 8.1.

It should be noted that several of the major types of metabolic myopathy are characterized histologically by major abnormalities in muscle fibres. For example, in those glycogenoses in which a myopathy is a feature glycogen is stored in muscle fibres; in the mitochondrial myopathies the mitochondria show characteristic abnormalities in number, distribution and ultrastructure (ragged-red fibres); in the lipid storage myopathies neutral lipid accumulates in muscle fibres; in the periodic paralyses, muscle fibres are often vacuolated in biopsies taken during a period of weakness.

Table 8.1 Metabolic myopathies: classified by their biochemical disorder (modified from Morgan-Hughes, 1989)

A. *Disorders of carbohydrate metabolism*
  (i)   Lysosomal glycogenolysis
         acid maltase deficiency (Type II glycogenosis)
  (ii) Glycogen synthesis
         branching enzyme deficiency (Type IV glycogenosis)
  (iii) Glycogenolysis
         debrancher enzyme deficiency (Type III glycogenosis)
         phosphorylase b kinase deficiency
         myophosphorylase deficiency (Type V glycogenosis:
         McArdle's disease)
  (iv) Glycolysis
         muscle phosphofructokinase deficiency (Type VII glycogenosis)
         phosphoglycerate kinase deficiency
         muscle phosphoglycerate mutase deficiency
         muscle lactate dehydrogenase deficiency

B. *Defects of mitochondrial metabolism*
  (i)   Substrate transport
         carnitine palmitoyl transferase deficiency
         primary carnitine deficiency
  (ii) Substrate utilization
         long-, medium- and short-chain acyl CoA dehydrogenase deficiencies
         multiple acyl CoA dehydrogenase deficiencies with electron transfer
         flavoprotein abnormalities
  (iii) Krebs' cycle defects
  (iv) Respiratory chain
         complex I deficiency (NADH CoQ reductase)
         complex II deficiency (succinate CoQ reductase)
         CoQ_{10} deficiency
         complex III deficiency (CoQ cytochrome C reductase)
         complex IV deficiency (cytochrome C oxidase)
         multiple respiratory enzyme defects
  (v)   Energy conservation
         Luft's disease
         ATP synthase deficiency

C. *Other muscle enzyme defects*
   myoadenylate deaminase deficiency

D. *Periodic paralysis* (disorders of muscle membrane Na/K transport)
   hypokalaemic, hyperkalaemic and normokalaemic periodic paralysis
   thyrotoxic periodic paralysis
   secondary hypokalaemic and hyperkalaemic muscular weakness

E. *Malignant hyperpyrexic myopathy*
   (neuroleptic malignant syndrome)

F. *Myoglobinurias* (see Table 8.2)

8.1.1   *Disorders of carbohydrate metabolism*

There are five main forms of glycogenosis associated with muscular involvement (Fig. 8.1).

(a) *Type II glycogenosis (acid maltase deficiency).* Two main forms of this disease occur. In the infantile form (Pompe's disease) there is generalized muscular weakness, with hypotonia, cardiomegaly and hepatomegaly, respiratory difficulties and enlargement of the tongue (Hogan *et al.*, 1969). The adult form resembles the limb-girdle dystrophy syndrome, presenting in adult life as a slowly progressive myopathy sometimes with calf hypertrophy (Engel, 1970a). An intermediate form, beginning in childhood, has also been described. The infantile and adult forms may occur in the same family (Busch *et al.*, 1979).

Muscle biopsy. The muscle fibres are rounded and show increased variability in size. There may be increased endomysial fibrous tissue. The major feature is the presence of PAS-positive vacuoles within muscle fibres. These vacuoles are usually multiple and very small. Their PAS-positive material is diastase-digestible and they are strongly reactive for acid phosphatase indicating that they are autophagic vacuoles derived from lysosomes (Engel, 1970a). In the adult form (Fig. 8.2) small angular fibres and fibre-type groupings, thought to indicate anterior horn cell involvement, have been reported (Karpati *et al.*, 1977). The biopsy is most abnormal in more severely affected muscles, and increased acid

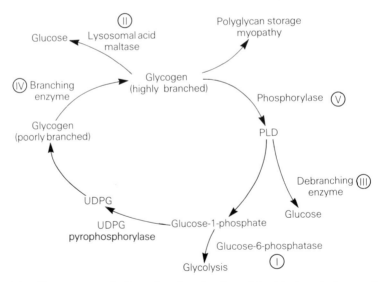

Fig. 8.1   Glycogen metabolism showing the sites of the biochemical errors in the five main types of glycogenosis.

phosphatase activity may be found in fibres apparently devoid of vacuoles (Swash *et al.*, 1985). In infantile cases all muscle fibres contain vacuoles. In ultrastructural studies most of the vacuoles are membrane bound or consist of autophagic vacuoles. Glycogen is found in both these sites, but is also present in increased quantity free in the sarcoplasm, between the myofibrils.

At autopsy relatively selective involvement of certain muscles, especially the diaphragm, is apparent. Minor abnormalities occur in smooth muscle of the gut and bladder. Cardiac muscle shows a gross vacuolar change with glycogen deposition in the infantile form and similar, but less marked, changes in the adult (van der Walt *et al.*, 1987). Involvement of the tongue is a feature in both forms of the disease.

(b) *Type III glycogenosis (debranching enzyme deficiency)*. In one form of the disease hepatomegaly, retardation of growth and attacks of hypoglycaemia are common but myopathy is slight, and in the other there is a prominent myopathy beginning in childhood or adult life, with progressive muscular weakness and hepatomegaly. Excessive fatiguability may be prominent (Brunberg *et al.*, 1971). There is electro-cardiographic evidence of cardiac involvement (Cornelio and DiDonato, 1985).

Muscle biopsy. There is a marked vacuolar myopathy. The vacuoles contain glycogen but are negative for acid phosphatase and the glycogen granules are not membrane bound. Sarcoplasmic glycogen is also increased. No neurogenic component has been reported (Di Mauro *et al.*, 1979).

(c) *Type IV glycogenosis (branching enzyme deficiency)*. Muscle weakness and atrophy is a mild feature of some patients with this disorder. Hepatosplenomegaly and failure to thrive are the main features. The disorder is extremely rare, affecting infants. An adult form probably also occurs (Ferguson *et al.*, 1983). The biopsy shows a vacuolar myopathy in which only scattered fibres are affected. Diaphragm and upper oesophagus are especially affected. Amylopectin (polysaccharide) deposits have been reported (McMaster *et al.*, 1979).

(d) *Type V glycogenosis (myophosphorylase deficiency)*. This is the commonest and the best known of the muscle glycogenoses (McArdle, 1951). The disorder may begin at any age but it is commonest in young adults. It presents with weakness, fatiguability and muscular cramps after exercise. Myoglobinuria may be a feature. At rest there is usually no clinical abnormality, although in long-standing cases muscular weakness and wasting may develop. Following ischaemic exercise there is little or no rise in the venous blood lactate or pyruvate levels. This abnormality is not specific for McArdle's disease since it is also found in phospho-fructokinase deficiency. Magnetic resonance spectroscopy studies show no reduction in intramuscular pH during anaerobic exercise, and a fall in creatine phosphate during aerobic exercise (Ross *et al.*, 1981). Glycogen accumulates because of the block in glycolysis. A severe infantile form has been reported (Di Mauro and Hartlage, 1978).

Muscle biopsy. Myophosphorylase is absent from the biopsy (Fig. 8.3), except in regenerating fibres in which the fetal form of the enzyme can be

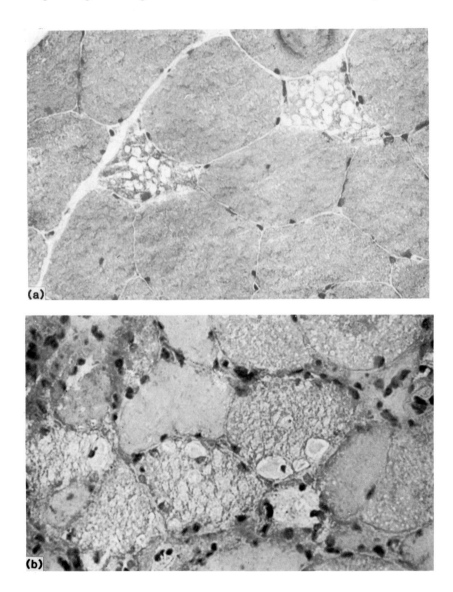

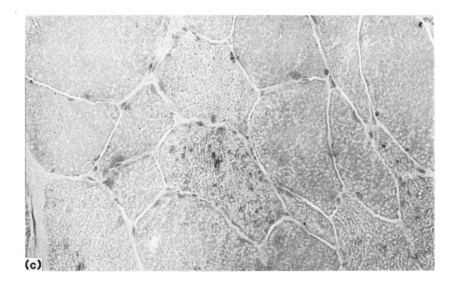

(c)

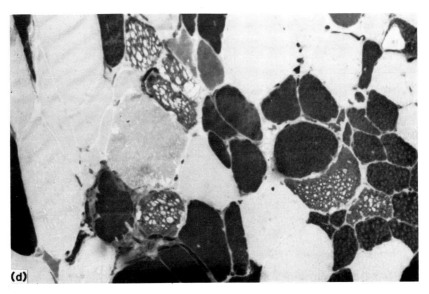

(d)

Fig. 8.2 Glycogen storage myopathy. (Type II glycogenosis; adult-onset type.) (a) × 350; HE. Two fibres show prominent vacuolization, and two contain central nuclei. (b) × 350; PAS. The vacuoles in the fibres (in another part of the biopsy) are PAS positive. (c) × 350; acid phosphatase. The vacuoles are filled with punctate positive reactivity indicative of lysosomal activity. (d) × 140; ATPase, pH 4.3. The vacuoles mainly affect fibres of intermediate type, but Type 2A fibres are also affected.

154   Metabolic, endocrine and drug-induced myopathies

detected (Di Mauro *et al.*, 1978). The muscle biopsy shows little other abnormality, apart from subsarcolemmal accumulations of PAS-positive glycogen, appearing as pink blebs (Fig. 8.4). Necrotic fibres, small atrophic fibres and scattered regenerating fibres may be prominent in

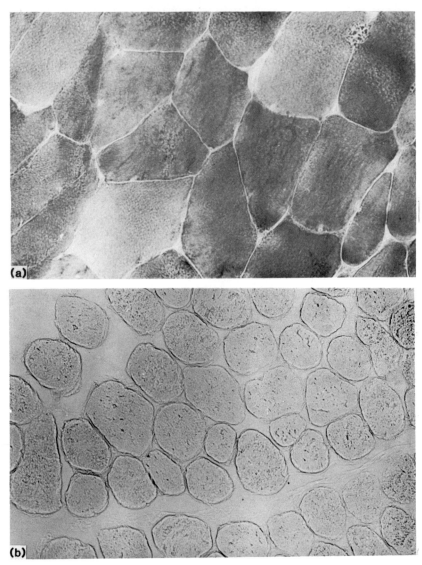

Fig. 8.3 McArdle's disease (Type V glycogenosis). (a) × 350. Myophosphorylase activity in normal muscle. (b) × 140. Absence of detectable myophosphorylase reactivity in McArdle's disease.

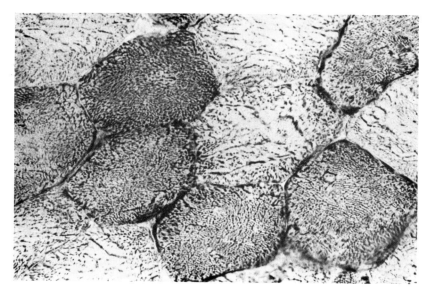

Fig. 8.4 McArdle's disease. × 350; PAS. There is unusually prominent glycogen, particularly in Type 1 fibres.

biopsies taken soon after severe exertion and in long-standing cases. There may be increased central nucleation (Dubowitz and Brooke, 1973). Ultrastructural studies show increased glycogen content in the intermyofibrillar sarcoplasm. It has been noted in some cases that individual muscles may show decreased, and others absent, phosphorylase activity. Smooth muscle is not involved, and the heart is also spared. Several different mutations have been recognized in myophosphorylase gene expression, resulting in variations in myophosphorylase content in different cases (Servidei *et al.*, 1988).

(e) *Type VII glycogenosis (phosphofructokinase deficiency)*. This rare disorder clinically resembles McArdle's disease, although muscular weakness is somewhat more prominent. The ischaemic exercise test is useful since, as in McArdle's disease, there is no rise in venous lactate or pyruvate after the period of ischaemic work. Red cell phosphofructokinase levels may be decreased and haemolytic disease has been noted (Tarui *et al.*, 1969).

Muscle biopsy. There is variation in fibre diameter, subsarcolemmal accumulation of glycogen, and a few necrotic fibres may be found (Tobin *et al.*, 1973). The absence of muscle phosphofructokinase can be demonstrated by an enzyme histochemical reaction (Bonilla and Schotland, 1970).

8.1.2   Defects of mitochondrial metabolism

The term mitochondrial myopathy has been used to describe a group of inherited disorders characterized by abnormalities in the morphology of mitochondria in muscle fibres, associated with metabolic errors affecting mitochondrial metabolism (Fig. 8.5). These disorders show maternal inheritance, since the mitochondrial genome is inherited from the mother. Similar morphological changes in mitochondria occur in patients with complex familial system degenerations of the nervous system, in which muscle involvement may occur. In these patients the clinical syndrome is determined by the distribution and severity of the biochemical disorder, rather than by its type (Petty *et al.*, 1986).

(a) *Clinical features.* Early-onset cases present with failure to thrive, hypotonia, seizures, mental retardation, ataxia and visual failure. Most infants with this syndrome have cytochrome C oxidase (complex IV) deficiency. Death occurs in metabolic acidosis with cardiorespiratory failure. There are later-onset presentations. Some patients present with progressive external ophthalmoplegia, often associated with mild proximal muscle weakness, and sometimes also with other features, e.g. cerebellar ataxia, cardiomyopathy with conduction block, retinal degeneration, mental retardation, sensory deafness and short stature (Kearns–Sayre syndrome; see Berenberg *et al.*, 1977). In others the clinical presentation is with slowly progressive proximal weakness, often without marked wasting, but usually with prominent fatiguability and reduced exercise tolerance. Muscle cramps, or even myoglobinuria, may be a feature. In the third group the CNS is involved, causing dementia,

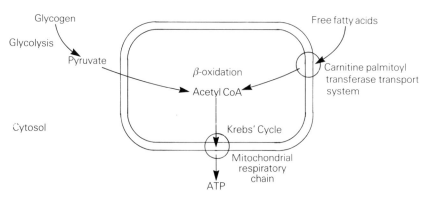

Fig. 8.5   Diagram of a single mitochondrion within the cytosol, showing free entry of pyruvate into the mitochondrial matrix. Free fatty acids cross the mitochondrial membrane utilizing a carnitine-dependent transport system. The respiratory chain system for ATP production is also located in the mitochondrial cristae.

deafness seizures, ataxia and involuntary movements. Two syndromes have been described; in MELAS there is mitochondrial encephalo-myopathy, lactic acidosis and strokes and in MERRF there is myoclonic epilepsy with ragged-red fibres (Berkovic *et al.*, 1989).

(b) *Pathological features.* Despite the various clinical presentations and the differing biochemical abnormalities most of these disorders show similar morphological changes in the muscle biopsy (Lombes *et al.*, 1989). The abnormality can almost invariably be recognized by light microscopy, without recourse to the electron microscope. The term ragged-red fibre is often used to describe the characteristic abnormality (Engel, 1971). Ragged-red fibres (Fig. 8.6) consist of fibres in which there is an irregular subsarcolemmal rim of bright red or reddish blue material in the Gomori trichrome stain. The abnormality is often patchily distributed through the cross-sectional area of the affected fibre. The abnormal material is positive in the oxidative enzyme reactions, e.g. NADH or SDH, faintly basophilic, usually positive for neutral lipid, and unreactive for ATPase. The most specific of these reactions is the SDH technique, since a positive reaction for this enzyme reaction is firm evidence for the presence of accumu-lations of mitochondria (Fig. 8.5). The ragged-red fibre abnormality particularly affects Type 1 muscle fibres (Olsen *et al.*, 1972), and these abnormal Type 1 fibres are almost always smaller than the unaffected Type 1 fibres. Generally there is little other abnormality, although there may be some increase in central nucleation, and some small angulated fibres and fibres showing a moth-eaten appearance in NADH reactions may be seen. Necrotic and regenerating fibres and interstitial fibrosis are not features of most of these disorders. However, a marked increase in the size and number of neutral lipid droplets, together with increased glycogen content, may be a prominent feature, especially in patients with muscle carnitine deficiency (Engel and Angelini, 1973). Lipid accumulates mainly in Type 1 fibres.

Although ragged-red fibres have come to be regarded as a specific feature of mitochondrial myopathies, in which they are prominent, occurring in as many as 20% of Type 1 fibres, single, isolated ragged-red fibres may sometimes be found in a variety of other disorders, e.g. polymyositis and limb-girdle dystrophy, in which a primary mito-chondrial disorder is not suspected. In order to suggest a diagnosis of mitochondrial myopathy ragged-red fibres should be the main patho-logical feature (Fig. 8.7), and other structural changes should be relatively minor (Olsen *et al.*, 1972).

With the electron microscope the mitochondrial abnormality can be further characterized (Tassin *et al.*, 1980). Subsarcolemmal and inter-myofibrillar aggregates of mitochondria are seen (Fig. 8.8). These mito-chondria are usually larger than normal, and abnormalities in their cristae

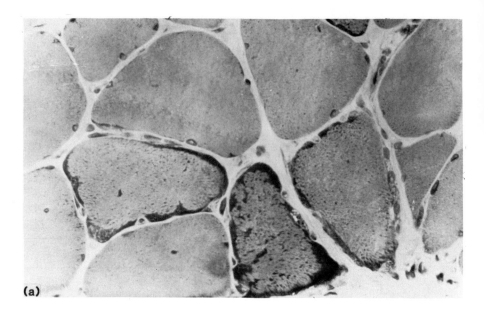

(a)

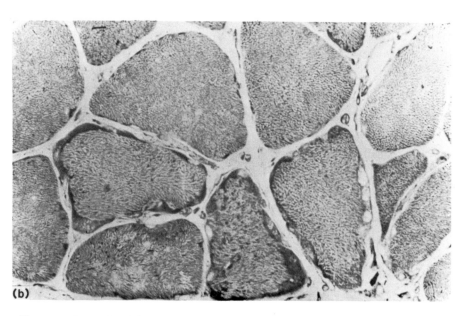

(b)

Fig. 8.6 Ragged-red fibres in a mitochondrial myopathy. × 600. (a) Gomori trichrome. The characteristic change is a peripheral, red-staining, zone, with a granular appearance to the fibre itself. (b) NADH. The peripheral zone is faintly positive with zones of non-reactivity. (c) ATPase, pH 4.3. The peripheral zone is non-reactive.

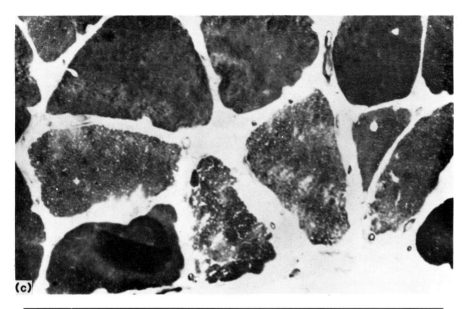

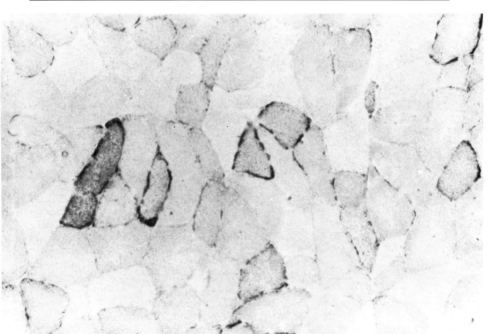

Fig. 8.7 Ragged-red fibres in cytochrome b deficiency. × 427; SDH. The mitochondrial-rich peripheral zone reacts darkly; the abnormal fibres are virtually all Type 1 fibres.

are prominent. Paracrystalline inclusions are particularly characteristic (Fig. 8.9), consisting of rectangular or curvilinear arrays of membranes arranged in a linear or grid-like pattern of about 20 nm separation. These inclusions are frequently multiple and arranged in parallel rows – the 'parking-lot' inclusions. They are usually situated between the displaced inner and outer membranes of the mitochondrion, and are often attached to these membranes by short, transverse bridges of membranous

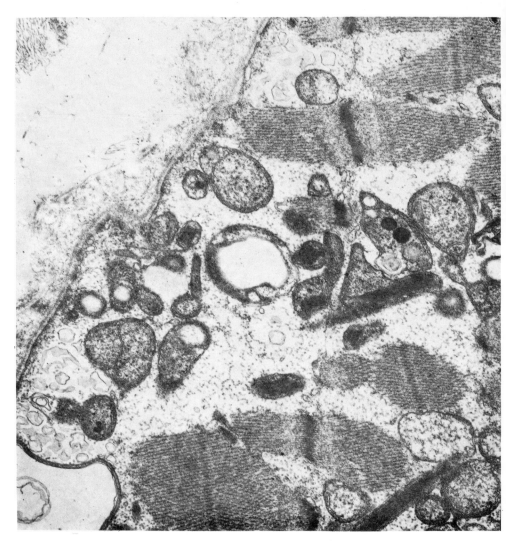

Fig. 8.8 Mitochondrial myopathy. Ragged-red fibres. EM, × 26 125. The mitochondria contain eosinophilic dense bodies, or paracrystalline material and their cristae are absent.

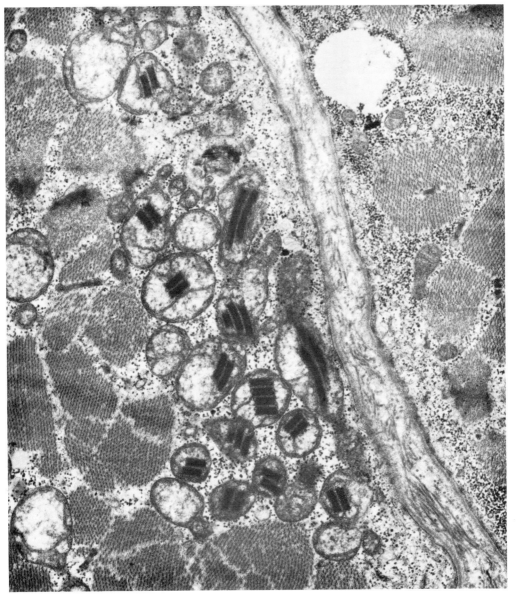

Fig. 8.9 EM, × 23 100. Paracrystalline inclusions in mitochondria in a ragged-red fibre.

material. Mitochondria containing paracrystalline inclusions are usually devoid of cristae. Other mitochondria show degraded cristae, or whorls of parallel membranes. Osmiophilic dense bodies and glycogen granules are also often found within the abnormal mitochondria in these disorders (Tassin and Brucher, 1982).

The myofibrillar architecture also shows abnormalities, with disarray or even fragmentation of myofibrils. There are increased amounts of sarcoplasmic glycogen, and lipid droplets are also unusually prominent.

(c) *Biochemical characterization.* The mitochondrial myopathies reflect the morphological expression of biochemical defects in metabolic pathways involving oxidative, mitochondrial-dependent processes (Di Mauro *et al.*, 1989). A number of genetically discrete abnormalities in mitochondrial metabolism have been characterized (Table 8.1). Ragged-red fibres are a feature of disorders of the respiratory chain, of disorders of substrate utilization, and of carnitine deficiency. In all these disorders the morphological abnormality, both by light and electron microscopy, has been similar to that described above. In carnitine deficiency muscle lipid droplet deposition is particularly prominent. Deletions of mitochondrial DNA have been recognized in a number of patients with mitochondrial encephalomyopathies (Holt *et al.*, 1988), and in some patients with progressive external ophthalmoplegia and Kearns–Sayre syndrome (Moraes *et al.*, 1989).

8.1.3   Lipid storage myopathies

This term has been used to describe accumulation of neutral lipid in muscle fibres. It is thus a non-specific abnormality. Lipid droplets occur in increased number in Type 1 muscle fibres in steroid myopathy and in alcoholic myopathy but they are particularly associated with defects of mitochondrial substrate transport or utilization (Table 8.1). The droplets consist of neutral lipid, predominantly triglycerides. Their distribution corresponds to the oxidative capacity of the muscle fibres so that lipid droplet accumulation is most marked in Type 1, less in Type 2A and least in Type 2B fibres. The droplets vary in size, are not membrane bound, and accumulate in the subsarcolemmal region and in rows between myofibrils. Lipid storage myopathy is usually associated with mito-chondrial abnormalities, reflecting the biochemical error in handling of mitochondrial substrate. These abnormalities consist of increased numbers or size of mitochondria, and the presence of intramitochondrial inclusions or changes in the morphology of the cristae.

Lipid storage myopathies are associated with carnitine deficiency. This may be a primary biochemical defect, or may occur secondary to defects of mitochondrial substrate utilization or to defects of intermediary metabolism associated with other disorders, e.g. renal failure, hypo-thyroidism, nutritional problems and cytochrome C oxidase deficiency.

Primary carnitine deficiency is an autosomal recessive disorder. In the adult form the disorder is limited to skeletal muscle, so that plasma and liver carnitine levels are normal. This disorder also occurs in children (Rebouche and Engel, 1983). Type 1 fibres are smaller than normal, and there are prominent neutral lipid droplets (Fig. 8.10) with mitochondrial abnormalities (Willner *et al.*, 1979). In childhood a severe systemic form of carnitine deficiency in which myopathy is associated with hepato-megaly, metabolic acidosis, hypoglycaemia, encephalopathy and cardio-myopathy, the muscle biopsy shows similar features to the adult-onset disorder (Karpati *et al.*, 1975). In carnitine palmitoyl transferase deficiency, a disorder presenting with cramps, muscular pain and myoglobinuria precipitated by exercise or fasting, the muscle biopsy shows little abnormality apart from a slight excess of lipid droplets in about 20% of cases (Bank *et al.*, 1975). Lipid droplets are also prominent in the mitochondrial myopathies themselves (see above). Some patients with carnitine deficiency respond to dietary supplementation with L-carnitine.

8.1.4   *Periodic paralysis*

This term refers to a group of disorders characterized by episodic and often asymmetrical limb-girdle weakness, sparing the respiratory muscles, with recovery between attacks. Attacks may last for several hours or days. Weakness occurs when the resting membrane potential is so low that the sodium channel is inactivated, preventing depolarization. There is usually an autosomal dominant pattern of inheritance. The commonest form is associated with *hypokalaemia* during attacks of weakness, but *hyperkalaemic* and *normokalaemic* forms have been described. In some patients a mild chronic proximal myopathy may develop.

In all three varieties of familial periodic paralysis the muscle biopsy shows only slight abnormalities between attacks but in biopsies taken shortly after an episode of weakness vacuolar change is prominent (Fig. 8.11). These membrane-bound vacuoles vary in size but do not deform the external shape of the fibre. They appear empty or faintly PAS positive. In patients who have sustained severe or prolonged weakness calcium salts may be deposited in the region of these vacuoles (Weller and McArdle, 1971). The vacuoles are unreactive for acid phosphatase, but affected fibres sometimes show faint or patchy basophilia. During the recovery phase the biopsy may contain a few necrotic fibres undergoing phagocytosis, and regenerating fibres may also be recognized.

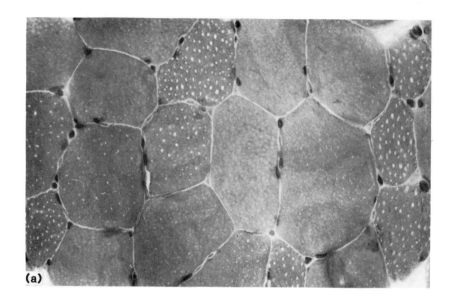

(a)

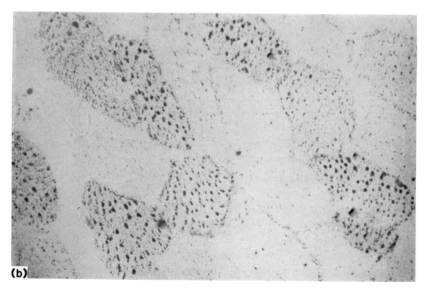

(b)

Fig. 8.10 Muscle carnitine deficiency of adult-onset. (a) × 350; HE. The striking abnormality is the presence of unstained, rounded lipid vacuoles of varying size, more prominent in some fibres than in others. These differ from ice crystals in their distribution, size and shape. (b) × 350; Oil red O. The vacuoles seen in the HE stain are stained intensely in this neutral lipid preparation. (c) × 350; ATPase, pH 4.3. The lipid droplets are unreactive, and are found mainly in Type 1 fibres.

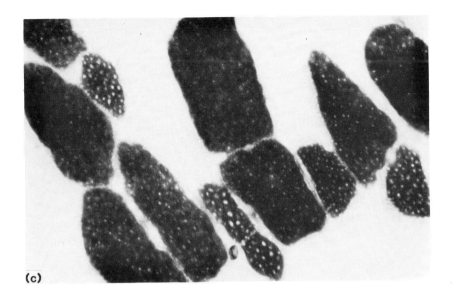

(c)

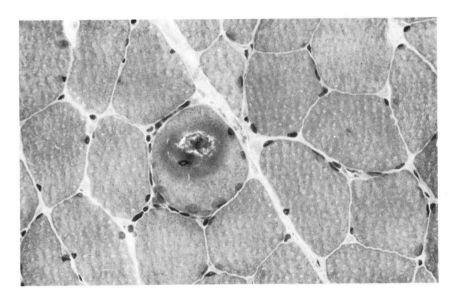

Fig. 8.11 Hypokalaemic periodic paralysis. × 350; HE. There is slight variability in fibre size with increased central nucleation. One fibre shows a prominent vacuolar zone, accompanied by central nucleation.

In patients in whom multiple attacks of weakness have occurred during many years, mild proximal weakness may be persistent and this is usually associated with histological features of a myopathy, including increased variability in fibre size, increased central nucleation and isolated necrotic and regenerating fibres, but even in these cases the presence of scattered vacuolated fibres should suggest the diagnosis.

Electron microscopy (Fig. 8.12) of vacuolated fibres reveals that the vacuoles, which are lined by a single layer of membrane, are continuous with dilated tubules of the sarcoplasmic reticulum (Engel, 1970b). The vacuoles often contain amorphous material, thought to consist of mucopolysaccharide. The sarcoplasm is normal but focal areas of myofibrillar disruption and repair are common. Similar vacuoles occur in other hypokalaemic myopathies, e.g. those associated with alcoholism (Rubenstein and Wainapel, 1977), liquorice toxicity, and diuretic abuse.

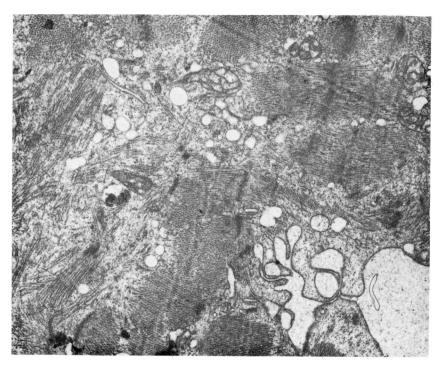

Fig. 8.12   EM. Hypokalaemic periodic paralysis. The origin of the vacuoles, lined by a single-layered membrane, from the tubular system can be seen. There is some disorganization of the myofibrillar pattern in this region.

8.1.5   Malignant hyperpyrexia myopathy and neuroleptic malignant syndrome

Although *malignant hyperpyrexia myopathy* is a metabolic myopathy the clinical features become apparent only after exposure to certain drugs, e.g. succinylcholine and anaesthetic drugs. The trait is inherited in an autosomal dominant pattern. The rapid rise in temperature that occurs during anaesthesia is accompanied by muscular rigidity, tachycardia and metabolic acidosis. There is massive myoglobinuria. Dantrolene therapy is effective, acting by decreasing calcium release from the sarcoplasmic reticulum (Morgan and Bryant, 1977). Susceptible individuals can sometimes be detected by the presence of a raised blood CK, but an *in vitro* test of muscle metabolism in the presence of low concentrations of anaesthetic agents, especially halothane, in which muscle contraction occurs in abnormal individuals, is far more reliable (Ellis and Halsall, 1980).

The muscle biopsy is usually abnormal; there are features of a mild non-progressive myopathy consisting of increased variability in fibre size, increased central nucleation, rare split fibres and some moth-eaten fibres. In some cases the histological features of central core disease have been reported (Denborough *et al.*, 1973). In acute episodes muscle fibre necrosis may be found, but there is often little abnormality apart from reduced glycogen content, a dilated tubular system and ruptured mitochondria (Schiller and Mair, 1974).

The *neuroleptic malignant syndrome* is an uncommon, idiosyncratic response to neuroleptic medication characterized by hyperpyrexia, muscular rigidity, impaired consciousness and elevated creatine kinase levels. In muscle samples taken during hyperpyrexia there is absence of glycogen and lipid droplets, and scattered muscle fibre necrosis, suggesting that heat production occurs from uncoupling of oxidative metabolism from contraction in muscle. A hypothalamic disturbance has also been suggested (Guze and Baxter, 1986; Martin and Swash, 1987).

8.1.6   Myoglobinurias

Generally, myoglobinuria is a feature associated with acute, massive muscle cell necrosis. It is therefore found in a wide variety of muscular disorders (Table 8.2). Myoglobin is a protein with a relatively low molecular weight (17 000 Dalton), and a low renal threshold. Urinary myoglobin reacts positively with benzidine, but can often be detected clinically by the characteristic brown colour. A sensitive immuno-precipitation method has recently supplanted the benzidine method (Markowitz and Wobig, 1977). Attacks of myoglobinuria are often

Table 8.2   Causes of myoglobinuria

Idiopathic paroxysmal myoglobinuria

Metabolic
    (a) Myophosphorylase deficiency (Glycogenosis Type V: McArdle's syndrome)
    (b) Phosphofructokinase deficiency (Glycogenosis Type VII)
    (c) Hypokalaemic periodic paralysis
    (d) Carnitine palmitoyl transferase deficiency
    (e) Malignant hyperpyrexia myopathy
    (f) Other systemic disorders, e.g. diabetic acidosis

Toxic
    (a) Alcohol, carbon monoxide and barbiturate poisoning
    (b) Liquorice excess (hypokalaemia)
    (c) Heroin myopathy
    (d) Chloroquine, amphotericin B and epsilon aminocaproic acid-induced acute toxic myopathies
    (e) Exposure to industrial toxins (Haff's disease)
    (f) Various biological toxins, e.g. hornet stings, Malaysian sea-snake bites, etc.
    (g) Heat stroke and high fever

Trauma and ischaemia
    (a) Crush injuries
    (b) Volkmann's ischaemic contracture
    (c) Anterior tibial syndrome ('shin splints')
    (d) Major arterial occlusion
    (e) Severe, prolonged exercise
    (f) Hyperosmolar states

Acute polymyositis and acute necrotizing myopathy associated with carcinoma

Postinfectious (viruses)
    (a) Influenza A
    (b) Coxsackie
    (c) *Herpes simplex*
    (d) Epstein–Barr

associated clinically with muscle weakness, pain and muscle swelling. In idiopathic myoglobinuria the attacks follow strenuous exercise, usually in young men (Type 1), or may be related to other unknown factors (Type 2).

The muscle biopsy in any myoglobinuric syndrome may show widespread acute muscle fibre necrosis. Regenerating fibres are often prominent, usually consisting of subsarcolemmal crescents of basophilic sarcoplasm of varying size, containing multiple lipid droplets. There may be a sparse lymphocytic infiltrate. The basic fascicular structure of the muscle is maintained, and histological recovery is usually complete unless recurrent attacks occur.

8.2   Endocrine myopathies

Myopathies are common features of endocrine disease (Table 8.3) but muscular involvement is comparatively rarely of clinical significance. Muscular symptoms may, however, be a presenting feature in hyper-thyroidism or in myxoedema, and sometimes also in disorders of calcium metabolism. Steroid myopathy is a common iatrogenic disorder, and a relatively late complication of Cushing's disease.

The CK may be greatly raised in some patients with myxoedema (McKeran *et al.*, 1980) although moderately increased levels are more common. In the other endocrine myopathies the CK is usually normal, although it may be slightly raised in some patients with acromegaly.

8.2.1   Muscle pathology

The histological changes in the muscle in endocrine myopathies are generally only slight, even when weakness is quite marked. In *acromegaly* Type 1 fibres are usually slightly hypertrophied and Type 2 fibres, especially Type 2A fibres, slightly atrophic (Nagulesparen *et al.*, 1976) but some hypertrophied Type 2 fibres may also be present. Necrotic muscle fibres are rarely seen (Mastaglia *et al.*, 1970). The muscle fibre hypertrophy may persist even after effective treatment of the acromegaly. In *hypo-* and *hyperparathyroidism* only minimal changes are found in the muscle; Type 2B atrophy has been noted in several studies (Schott and Wills, 1975). The morphological changes in osteomalacia are similarly slight.

Table 8.3   Endocrine myopathies

Thyroid myopathies
  Hyperthyroidism
  Hypothyroidism

Parathyroid disorders and osteomalacia
  Hypoparathyroidism
  Hyperparathyroidism
  Osteomalacia

Adrenal disorders (and steroid myopathy)
  Addison's disease
  Cushing's syndrome
  Steroid therapy

Pituitary disorders
  Acromegaly
  Hypopituitarism

In *hyperthyroidism* the main abnormality is atrophy of muscle fibres, but this may be very slight. Focal lymphocytic infiltrates may be present. Muscle fibre necrosis is not a feature, but central nucleation may be excessive. In *myxoedema* light microscopy may reveal some fibre atrophy, increased central nucleation and occasional fibres with subsarcolemmal accumulation of glycogen (McKeran *et al.*, 1980). Degenerating and regenerating fibres are rare (Shirabe *et al.*, 1975). Ultrastructural studies have revealed accumulation of abnormal mitochondria, some containing rectilinear paracrystalline bodies similar to those found in primary mitochondrial myopathies (Godet-Guillain and Fardeau, 1970).

Steroid myopathy shows more marked abnormalities in the muscle biopsy. The main feature is atrophy of both fibre types, particularly of Type 2B fibres (Pleasure *et al.*, 1970). Lipid droplets and glycogen accumulations are prominent, especially in Type 1 fibres. Electron microscopy shows enlarged and degenerate mitochondria, dilatation of the sarcoplasmic reticulum, loss of myofibrils and marked thickening of the basement membrane (Engel, 1966). In the light microscope the Type 2 fibre atrophy may be so prominent that the presence of scattered atrophic fibres in the HE preparation may be interpreted as denervation (Fig. 8.13); however, the limitation of this atrophy to Type 2 fibres in the enzyme histochemical preparation rules out this possibility (Fig. 8.14).

Muscle biopsies are sometimes used to try to assess the possible

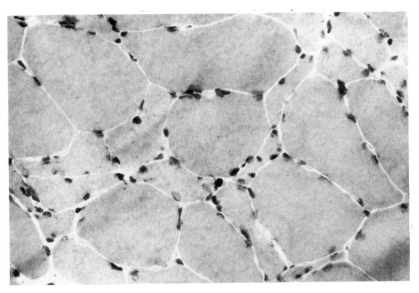

Fig. 8.13   Steroid myopathy. × 350; HE. There is atrophy of some fibres.

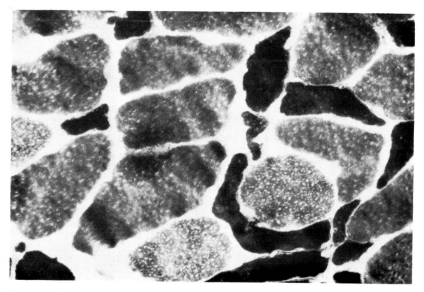

Fig. 8.14   Steroid myopathy. × 350; ATPase, pH 9.4. The atrophic fibres are all Type 2 fibres. The paler Type 1 fibres are much less affected.

development of steroid myopathy in patients with polymyositis who have been treated with high-dose steroids for some weeks, yet have remained weak, or even become weaker during treatment. The presence of lipid-laden fibres, especially Type 1 fibres, and of Type 2B fibre atrophy, strongly suggest that steroid myopathy has developed (Askari *et al.*, 1976). The dose of steroid necessary to induce steroid myopathy is variable, e.g. 1.5–6.0 mg dexamethasone daily for 3–12 weeks, and prednisone 15–100 mg daily for periods ranging from 1 month to 5 years (Afifi *et al.*, 1968; Askari *et al.*, 1976).

8.3   Drug-induced myopathies

A large number of different drugs may cause muscular weakness (Swash and Schwartz, 1983). *Painful* proximal myopathies, sometimes associated with myoglobinuria, or with a raised blood CK level, may occur acutely or subacutely. Examples include myopathies associated with alcoholism (Fig. 8.15), emetine and epsilon aminocaproic acid treatment. A chronic *painless* myopathy has been described after treatment with chloroquine, perhexilene and steroids, and a similar syndrome may occur in opiate addiction. Repeated intramuscular injection may cause a *focal* myopathy, usually associated with intense local fibrosis. Penicillamine may induce

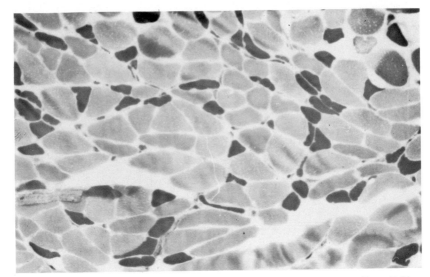

Fig. 8.15 Alcoholic myopathy. × 140; ATPase, pH 9.4. Prominent Type 2 fibre atrophy.

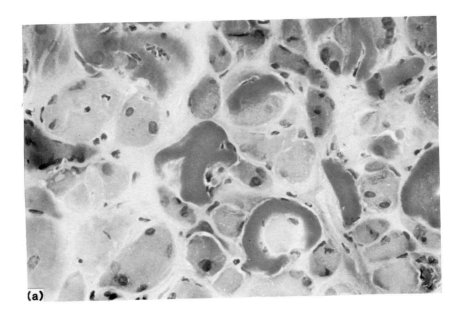

(a)

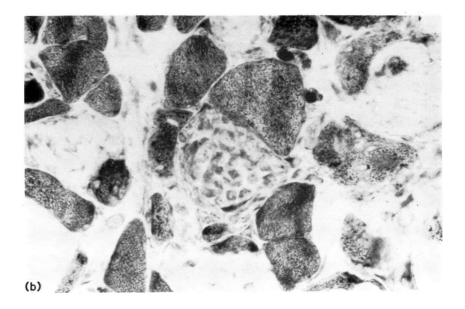

(b)

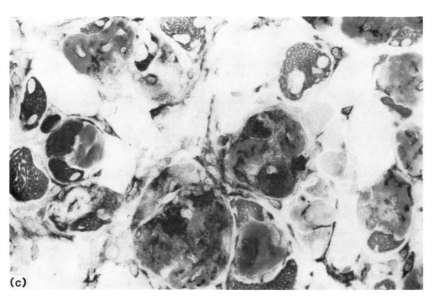

(c)

Fig. 8.16 Epsilon aminocaproic acid myopathy: an acute necrotizing 'toxic' myopathy. (a) × 450; HE. The field consists of necrotic muscle fibres, with peripheral crescents of regeneration. There is a sparse inflammatory cell exudate. (b) × 450; NADH. The regenerating segments are clearly seen in this part of the biopsy. (c) × 450; ATPase, pH 4.3. The regenerating segments show ATPase reactivity, but the necrotic portions of these fibres are unreactive.

174   Metabolic, endocrine and drug-induced myopathies

myasthenia gravis or inflammatory myopathy. Hypokalaemia and vacuolar myopathy may follow treatment with diuretics or purgatives.

In the acute and subacute myopathies fibre necrosis and regeneration may be prominent (Fig. 8.16), and myopathic features may be present in the more chronic drug-induced myopathies. Both perhexilene and chloroquine may cause a vacuolar myopathy. The drug-induced neuromuscular syndromes have been reviewed by Mastaglia and Argov (1981).

References

Afifi, A.K., Bergman, R.A. and Harvey, J.C. (1968) Steroid myopathy: clinical, histological and cytological observations. *Johns Hopkins Med. J.*, **123**, 158–174.
Askari, A., Vignos, P.J. Jr. and Moskowitz, R.W. (1976) Steroid myopathy in connective tissue diseases. *Am. J. Med.*, **61**, 485–492.
Bank, W.J., Di Mauro, S., Bonilla, E. *et al.* (1975) A disorder of lipid metabolism and myoglobinuria. *N. Engl. J. Med.*, **292**, 443–449.
Berenberg, R.A., Pellock, J.M., Di Mauro, S. *et al.* (1977) Lumping or splitting? 'Opthalmoplegia plus' or Kearns–Sayre syndrome? *Ann. Neurol.*, **1**, 37–54.
Berkovic, S.F., Carpenter, S., Evans, A. *et al.* (1989) Myoclonus epilepsy and ragged-red fibres (MERRF), *Brain*, **112**, 1231–1260.
Bonilla, E. and Schotland, D.L. (1970) Histochemical diagnosis of muscle phosphofructokinase deficiency. *Arch. Neurol.*, **22**, 8–12.
Brunberg, J.A., McCormick, W.F. and Schochet, S.S. (1971) Type III glycogenosis. An adult with diffuse weakness and muscle wasting. *Arch. Neurol.*, **25**, 171–178.
Busch, H.F.M., Koster, J.F. and van Weerden, T.W. (1979) Infantile and adult-onset acid maltase deficiency occurring in the same family. *Neurology*, **29**, 415–416.
Cornelio, F. and Di Donato, S. (1985) Myopathies due to enzyme deficiencies. *J. Neurol.*, **232**, 329–340.
Denborough, M.A., Dennett, X. and Anderson, P.M. (1973) Central core disease and malignant hyperpyrexia. *Br. Med. J.*, **1**, 272–273.
Di Mauro, S. and Hartlage, P.L. (1978) Fatal infantile form of muscle phosphorylase deficiency. *Neurology*, **28**, 1124–1129.
Di Mauro, S., Arnold, S., Miranda, A. and Rowland, L.P. (1978) McArdle's disease: the mystery of reappearing phosphorylase activity in muscle culture – a fetal isoenzyme. *Ann. Neurol.*, **3**, 60–66.
Di Mauro, S., Bonilla, E., Zeviani, M. *et al.* (1989) Mitochondrial myopathies. *J. Inherit. Metab. Dis.*, **10**, Suppl. 1, 113–128.
Di Mauro, S., Hartwig, G.B., Hayes, A. *et al.* (1979) Debranching enzyme deficiency: neuromuscular disorders in 5 adults. *Ann. Neurol.*, **5**, 422–436.
Dubowitz, V. and Brooke, M.H. (1973) *Muscle Biopsy – A Modern Approach*, W.B. Saunders, London.
Ellis, F.R. and Halsall, P.J. (1980) Malignant hyperpyrexia. *Br. J. Hosp. Med.*, **24**, 318–327.
Engel, A.G. (1966) Electron microscopic observations in thyrotoxic and corticosteroid-induced myopathies. *Mayo Clin. Proc.*, **41**, 785–796.
Engel, A.G. (1970a) Acid maltase deficiency in adults. *Brain*, **93**, 599–606.
Engel, A.G. (1970b) Evolution and content of vacuoles in primary hypokalemic periodic paralysis. *Mayo Clin. Proc.*, **45**, 774–814.

Engel, A.G. and Angelini, C. (1973) Carnitine deficiency of human muscle with associated lipid storage myopathy: a new syndrome. *Science*, **179**, 899–902.

Engel, W.K. (1971) 'Ragged-red fibres' in ophthalmoplegia syndromes and their differential diagnosis. In *Muscle Diseases* (ed. B.A. Kakulas), ICS 237, Excerpta Medica, Amsterdam, p. 28.

Ferguson, I.T., Mahon, M. and Cumming, W.J.K. (1983) An adult case of Andersen's disease: Type IV glycogenosis. *J. Neurol. Sci.*, **60**, 337–351.

Godet-Guillain, J. and Fardeau, M. (1970) Hypothyroid myopathy: histological and ultrastructural study of an atrophic form. In *Muscle Diseases* (eds J.N. Walton, N. Canal and S. Scarlato), ICS 199, Excerpta Medica, Amsterdam, pp. 512–515.

Guze, B.H. and Baxter, L.R. (1986) Neuroleptic malignant syndrome. *N. Engl. J. Med.*, **313**, 163–166.

Hogan, G.R., Gutamann, L., Schmidt, R. and Gilbert, E. (1969) Pompe's disease. *Neurology*, **19**, 894–900.

Holt, I.J., Harding, A.E. and Morgan-Hughes, J.A. (1988) Deletions of mitochondrial DNA in patients with mitochondrial myopathies. *Nature*, **331**, 717–719.

Karpati, G., Carpenter, S., Engel, A.G. *et al.* (1975) The syndrome of systemic carnitine deficiency . *Neurology*, **25**, 16–24.

Karpati, G., Carpenter, S., Eisen, A. *et al.* (1977) The adult form of acid maltase (α1 : 4 glucosidase) deficiency. *Ann. Neurol.*, **1**, 276–280.

Lombes, A., Bonilla, E. and Di Mauro, S. (1989) Mitochondrial encephalomyopathies. *Rev. Neurol.*, **145**, 671–689.

McArdle, B. (1951) Myopathy due to a defect in muscle glycogen breakdown. *Clin. Sci.*, **10**, 13–33.

McKeran, R.O., Slavin, G., Ward, P. *et al.* (1980) Hypothyroid myopathy: a clinical and pathological study. *J. Pathol.*, **132**, 35–54.

McMaster, K.R., Powers, J.M., Hennigar, G.R. *et al.* (1979) Nervous system involvement in Type IV glycogenosis. *Arch. Pathol. Lab. Med.*, **103**, 105–111.

Markowitz, H. and Wobig, G.H. (1977) Quantitative method for estimating myoglobin in urine. *Clin. Chem.*, **23**, 1689–1693.

Martin, D.T. and Swash, M. (1987) Muscle pathology in the neuroleptic malignant syndrome. *J. Neurol.*, **235**, 120–121.

Mastaglia, F.L. and Argov, Z. (1981) Drug-induced neuromuscular disorders in man. In *Disorders of Voluntary Muscle*, 4th edn (ed. J.N. Walton), Churchill Livingstone, Edinburgh, pp. 873–906.

Mastaglia, F.L., Barwick, D.D. and Hall, R. (1970) Myopathy in acromegaly. *Lancet*, **2**, 907–909.

Moraes, C.T., Di Mauro, S., Zeviani, M. *et al.* (1989) Mitochondrial DNA deletions in progressive external ophthalmoplegia and Kearns–Sayre syndrome. *N. Engl. J. Med.*, **320**, 1293–1299.

Morgan, K.G. and Bryant, S.H. (1977) The mechanism of action of dantrolene sodium. *J. Pharmacol. Exp. Ther.*, **201**, 138–141.

Morgan-Hughes, J.A. (1989) The metabolic myopathies. *Curr. Opin. Neurol. Neurosurg.*, **2**, 689–694.

Nagulesparen, M., Trickey, R., Davies, M.J. and Jenkins, J.S. (1976) Muscle changes in acromegaly. *Br. Med. J.*, **2**, 914–915.

Olson, W., Engel, W.K., Walsh, G.O. and Einaugler, R. (1972) Oculo-craniosomatic neuromuscular disease with 'ragged-red fibres'. Histochemical and ultrastructural changes in limb muscles of a group of patients with idiopathic progressive external ophthalmoplegia. *Arch. Neurol.*, **26**, 193–211.

Petty, R.K.H., Harding, A.E. and Morgan-Hughes, J.A. (1986) The clinical features of mitochondrial myopathy. *Brain*, **109**, 915–938.

Pleasure, D.E., Walsh, G.O. and Engel, W.K. (1970) Atrophy of skeletal muscles in patients with Cushing's syndrome. *Arch. Neurol.*, **22**, 118–125.

Rebouche, C.J. and Engel, A.G. (1983) Carnitine metabolism and deficiency syndromes. *Mayo Clin. Proc.*, **58**, 533–540.

Ross, B.D., Radda, G.K., Godian, D.G. *et al.* (1981) Examination of a case of suspected McArdle's syndrome by ^{31}P nuclear magnetic resonance. *N. Engl. J. Med.*, **304**, 1338–1342.

Rubenstein, A.E. and Wainapel, S.F. (1977) Acute hypokalemic myopathy in alcoholism. *Arch. Neurol.*, **34**, 553–555.

Schiller, H.H. and Mair, W.G.P. (1974) Ultrastructural changes of muscle in malignant hyperthermia. *J. Neurol. Sci.*, **21**, 93–100.

Schott, G.D. and Wills, M.R. (1975) Myopathy in hypophosphataemic osteomalacia presenting in adult life. *J. Neurol. Neurosurg. Psychiatry*, **38**, 297–304.

Servidei, S., Shanske, S., Zeviani, M. *et al.* (1988) McArdle's disease: biochemical and molecular genetic studies. *Ann. Neurol.*, **24**, 774–781.

Shirabe, T., Tawara, S., Terao, A. and Araki, S. (1975) Myxoedematous polyneuropathy. *J. Neurol. Neurosurg. Psychiatry*, **38**, 241–247.

Swash, M. and Schwartz, M.S. (1983) Iatrogenic neuromuscular disorders: a review. *Proc. R. Soc. Med.*, **76**, 149–151.

Swash, M., Schwartz, M.S. and Apps, M.C.P. (1985) Adult-onset acid maltase deficiency. *J. Neurol. Sci.*, **68**, 61–74.

Tarui, S., Kono, N., Nasu, T. and Nishikawa, M. (1969) Enzymatic basis for the co-existence of myopathy and hemolytic disease in inherited muscle phosphofructokinase deficiency. *Biochem. Biophys. Res. Comm.*, **34**, 77–83.

Tassin, S. and Brucher, J.M. (1982) The mitochondrial disorders: pathogenesis and aetiological classification. *Neuropathol. Appl. Neurobiol.*, **8**, 251–263.

Tassin, S., Walter, G.F., Brucher, J.M. and Rousseau, J.J. (1980) Histochemical and ultrastructural analysis of the mitochondrial changes in a familial mitochondrial myopathy. *Neuropathol. Appl. Neurobiol.*, **6**, 227–247.

Tobin, W.E., Hijing, F., Porro, R.S. and Salzman, R.T. (1973) Muscle phosphofructokinase deficiency. *Arch. Neurol.*, **28**, 128–130.

Van der Walt, J.D., Swash, M., Leake, J. and Cox, E.L. (1987) The pattern of involvement of adult-onset acid maltase deficiency at autopsy. *Muscle Nerve*, **10**, 272–281.

Weller, R.O. and McArdle, B. (1971) Calcification within muscle fibres in the periodic paralyses. *Brain*, **94**, 263–272.

Willner, J., Di Mauro, S., Eastwood, A. *et al.* (1979) Muscle carnitine deficiency: genetic heterogeneity. *J. Neurol. Sci.*, **41**, 235–246.

9 Neurogenic disorders

The neurogenic disorders include diseases affecting anterior horn cells, nerve roots and peripheral nerves. In many of these there is involvement of neural pathways, other than the lower motor neuron. For example, in motor neuron disease there is almost always involvement of the upper motor neuron and in peripheral neuropathies sensory fibres are also involved. In this chapter only the changes seen in muscle biopsies will be described. A general account of the pathology of these disorders is given in other texts (e.g. Weller *et al.*, 1983). In many neurogenic disorders muscle biopsy is not indicated but in children muscle biopsy is useful in the diagnosis of spinal muscular atrophies and in adults, muscle biopsies are sometimes used in motor neuron disease when there is doubt about the diagnosis, particularly in patients with bulbar palsy without evident clinical involvement of the limbs. Sometimes muscle biopsies of adults with chronic neurogenic disorders are carried out to exclude polymyositis.

The blood CK level is usually normal in neurogenic disorders, but confusion may arise in chronic conditions, especially in Kugelberg–Welander disease, in chronic motor neuropathies, e.g. Charcot–Marie–Tooth disease, and in motor neuron disease, since in these neurogenic disorders the CK may be raised to as much as ten times above normal. This is often accompanied by the development of secondary changes of myopathic type (Schwartz *et al.*, 1976).

9.1 Spinal muscular atrophies

This group of disorders consists of a clinical syndrome of proximal muscular weakness and wasting of varying age of onset, progression and severity. They are inherited as autosomal recessive traits; sporadic cases are common. Several different forms are recognized, as listed in Table 9.1.

Weakness is often predominantly proximal especially in the late-onset form, e.g. Type 3 spinal muscular atrophy and, although the disorder is neurogenic in origin, the clinical features of the lower neuron lesion may

Table 9.1   Spinal muscular atrophies

	Age of onset	Outcome
Type 1 (Werdnig–Hoffmann disease)	Usually before 3 months	95% dead by age 18 months
Type 2 (Intermediate form)	6–12 months	Variable life expectancy, severe disability
Type 3 (Kugelberg–Welander disease)	2–15 years	Normal life expectancy, mild or moderate disability
Type 4 (Adult onset)	15–50 years	Mild disability

be difficult to recognize. For example, fasciculation is often not present at rest. As a result these disorders are easily mistaken for myopathies and the finding of neurogenic change in the muscle biopsy may be unexpected. Other less common clinical syndromes of spinal muscular atrophy are recognized, including distal, asymmetrical, bulbar and facioscapulohumeral types.

9.1.1   Muscle biopsy

The pathological features differ in the four main forms of spinal muscular atrophy, probably because of the effects of immaturity of the neuro-muscular system in the Type 1 and Type 2 forms.

In *Werdnig–Hoffmann disease* (Type 1 spinal muscular atrophy) the characteristic feature is the presence of large groups of small rounded atrophic fibres, which may encompass the whole fascicle. In addition, hypertrophied fibres, often three or four times normal size, are found intermingled with the atrophic fibres, and interfascicular fibrosis may be prominent (Fig. 9.1a,b). The rounded atrophic fibres may be of either fibre type, and may show fibre-type grouping of variable degree. The hypertrophied fibres are usually Type 1 fibres in ATPase preparations (Fig. 9.1c) but they show variable NADH reactivity suggesting that they have mixed histochemical characteristics. Other structures, for example nerves, blood vessels and muscle spindles, appear normal. Indeed, muscle spindles may appear unusually prominent because they are relatively resistant to denervation atrophy and thus are relatively preserved amidst the sheets of atrophic fibres so characteristic of the disease. Motor end-plates appear atrophic, and the terminal axons beaded and tortuous.

The abnormality in the muscle biopsy in Type 1 spinal muscular atrophy varies according to the duration of the disease and the muscle biopsied. In particular, hypertrophied fibres may be absent, or less prominent, in biopsies taken in the first few weeks of life (Fig. 9.1d,e), but may appear a few months later (Dubowitz, 1978). The origin of these hypertrophied fibres thus relates to developmental factors, possibly to work hypertrophy; as muscles come to be used during development, the few remaining fibres are required to carry out normal tasks. In addition, spontaneous EMG activity has been recorded in this disease and this may be a factor leading to hypertrophy (see Swash and Schwartz, 1988). The atrophic fibres resemble immature, fetal muscle fibres in their histochemical and ultrastructural features and thus may represent maturational arrest, occurring as a result of lack of development of normal innervation (Hausmanowa-Petrusiewicz *et al.*, 1980). The presence of these fetal fibres may prevent the orderly innervation and maturation of other muscle fibres within the muscle.

Intermediate spinal muscular atrophy (Type 2) is uncommon. The muscle biopsy resembles that of Werdnig–Hoffman disease, but fibre-type grouping is more prominent, including groups of small atrophic fibres, fibres of normal size and hypertrophied fibres (Fig. 9.2). Separate fascicles vary greatly in the degree of abnormality. Angulated fibres, characteristic of denervation in mature muscle, are not found in Type 2 or Type 1 spinal muscular atrophy. The severity of the changes in the muscle biopsy in Type 2 spinal muscular atrophy is not a reliable indicator of prognosis (Dubowitz and Brooke, 1973). In some biopsies in this condition, especially in older children who have entered a clinically stable phase of the disease, increased central nucleation and fibre splitting, indicative of secondary myopathic change, may occur but this is usually mild. Sometimes core fibres and target fibres may occur.

Kugelberg–Welander disease (Type 3 spinal muscular atrophy) is the commonest form of this group of disorders. It may be clinically indistinguishable from proximal myopathy or limb-girdle muscular dystrophy and muscle biopsies often show prominent myopathic abnormalities, especially in older patients. These myopathic changes consist of degenerative and regenerative changes in individual fibres, muscle fibre splitting, hypertrophy and atrophy of fibres leading to abnormal variation in fibre size, central nucleation and endomysial and interfascicular fibrosis. Indeed, in HE preparations (Fig. 9.3), whether of formalin-fixed or frozen material, the biopsy may show such marked myopathic change, that the presence of the primary underlying neurogenic disorder may be missed. Enzyme histochemical studies, however, are diagnostic, since they reveal fibre-type grouping (Fig. 9.4). The groups consist of small groups of fibres of either histochemical type. The fibres in these groups are usually of normal size. In some biopsies

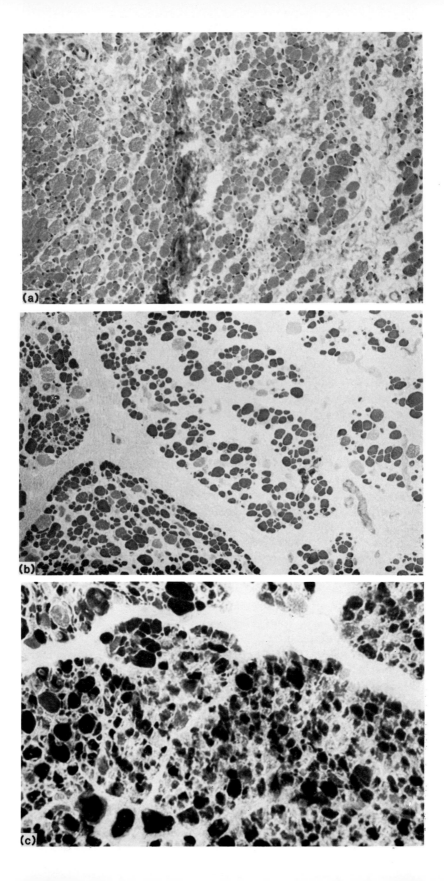

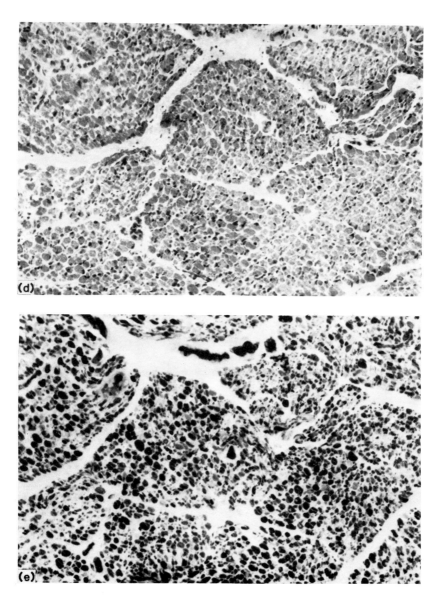

Fig. 9.1 Werdnig–Hoffmann disease. (a) × 140; HE. Fibrosis and loss of muscle fibres with hypertrophy of some of the remaining fibres are the major features. There are many tiny (< 10 μm) round fibres. (b) × 140; ATPase, pH 9.5. Perimysial thickening, loss of muscle fibres, and hypertrophy of both fibre types are prominent. There are many small rounded fibres and the distribution of atrophic and hypertrophied fibres is similar in the three fascicles illustrated. Fibre-type grouping is not a feature. (c) × 350; ATPase, pH 4.5. The hypertrophied fibres are darkly reactive Type 1 fibres. (d) × 140; HE. In this biopsy from an infant aged 2 weeks, fibre hypertrophy is not prominent although there are many areas of very small rounded fibres. (e) × 140; ATPase, pH 4.5. There is no fibre-type grouping, and fibrosis is not a feature. A few larger fibres are darkly reactive, but most fibres are atrophic.

some fascicles contain small, pointed, NADH-dark, atrophic fibres, whereas adjoining fascicles consist of fibres of normal size, arranged in the pattern of fibre-type grouping. The presence of these denervated atrophic fibres indicates failure of compensatory reinnervation, that is ineffective collateral sprouting, whereas the fibre-type groups represent effective reinnervation from collateral sprouting. The former may indicate that the disease is likely to be progressive. In many biopsies very large fibres, up to 150 μm diameter, may be seen. These are thought to result from work hypertrophy (Swash and Schwartz, 1977), and are particularly likely to show fibre splitting if examined in serial transverse sections.

Small, rounded atrophic fibres, similar to those found in Werdnig–Hoffmann disease, may also be found in Type 3 spinal muscular atrophy, suggesting that this disorder may also begin in infancy, although clinical presentation is delayed until childhood or adolescence.

Adult-onset spinal muscular atrophy (Type 4) shows similar changes to those found in Kugelberg–Welander disease. Various other atypical forms have been reported. These include distal spinal muscular atrophy, patients with focal and non-progressive involvement of one limb, and

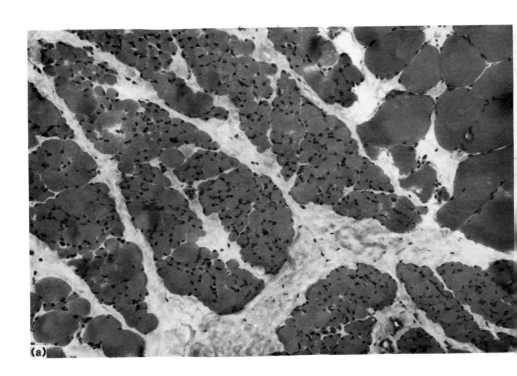

(a)

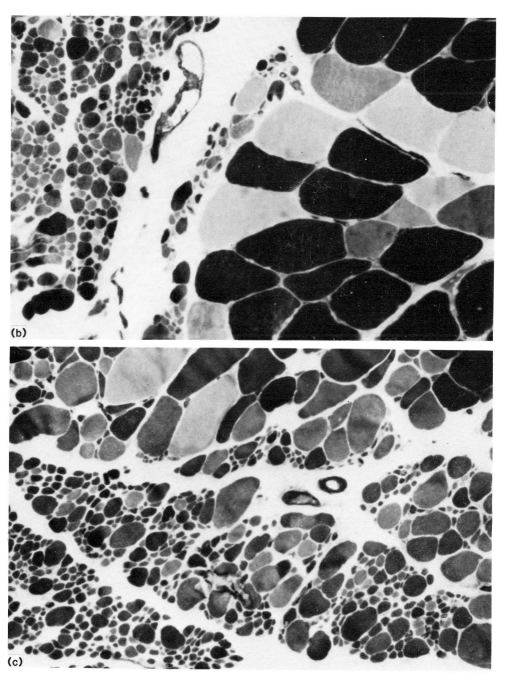

Fig. 9.2 Intermediate (Type 2) spinal muscular atrophy. Child aged 6 years. (a) × 380; HE. There are sheets of small rounded fibres of slightly varying size occupying several fascicles: a nearby fascicle consists of larger fibres. The perimysium is thickened. (b) × 380; ATPase, pH 4.5. The small fibres vary in histochemical type and size. (c) × 380; ATPase, pH 4.5. The demarcation between the small and the larger fibres is not necessarily abrupt or at a fascicular boundary.

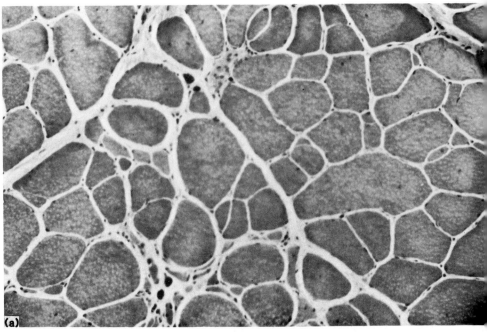

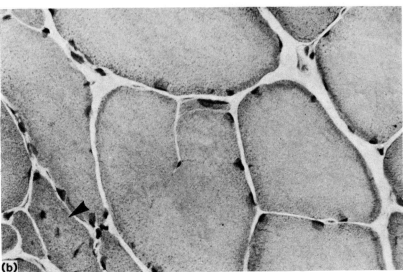

Fig. 9.3 Kugelberg–Welander disease (Type 3 spinal muscular atrophy). (a) × 133; HE. There is markedly increased variation in fibre size and fibre splitting with increased central nucleation and increased endomysial and perimysial connective tissue. These are myopathic features, but the underlying neurogenic features are apparent only in ATPase preparations. (b) × 560; HE. Fibre-splitting is associated with central nucleation, or with regeneration as in the smaller granular fibre (arrow).

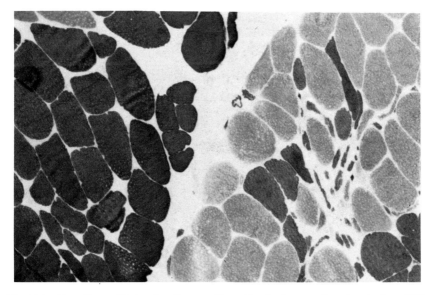

Fig. 9.4   Kugelberg–Welander disease (Type 3 spinal muscular atrophy). × 140; ATPase, pH 4.3. There is type grouping of both Type 1 and Type 2 fibres, and the groups are very large, indicating effective reinnervation. Several clusters of small pointed denervated fibres are also present. The variability in fibre size within the fibre grouping is apparent.

others with a scapuloperoneal pattern of weakness. These rare disorders show similar pathological features to those of Type 3 spinal muscular atrophy and thus form clinical syndromes without specific pathological features.

Autopsy findings in spinal muscular atrophies are incompletely documented. In all the main types there is widespread loss of anterior horn cells, with end-stage denervation and atrophy of the limb and girdle musculature. In Werdnig–Hoffmann disease there is also loss of motor neutrons in the bulbar nuclei, with particularly severe loss of lumbar anterior horn cells (Marshall and Duchen, 1975). In Type 3 spinal muscular atrophy loss of anterior horn cells is less marked than in the Type 1 disorder, and bulbar motoneurons appear unaffected (Tomlinson *et al.*, 1974).

9.2   Motor neuron disease

This progressive and almost invariably fatal disease is usually readily diagnosed by clinical investigation. Presentation is usually as a mixed upper and lower motor neuron disorder, with weakness, atrophy, fasciculations and brisk tendon reflexes, but bulbar and lower motor neuron forms may occur and occasionally other atypical presentations such as primary ventilatory failure may lead to muscle biopsy. Asymmetrical involvement of the limbs is common and may be difficult to distinguish from the effects of vertebral spondylosis with root lesions. Median survival is 3 years from the onset of the disease, although some 20% of cases may survive for longer than 5 years.

9.2.1   Muscle biopsy

Three interrelated types of abnormality in this progressive disorder can be recognized (Table 9.2). These can be correlated with the stage of the disease, and the extent of compensatory reinnervation and other compensatory processes, e.g. fibre hypertrophy and fibre splitting.

The most prominent abnormality is the presence of small angulated fibres, often found in small clusters (Fig. 9.5). These fibres may be of either histochemical type (Fig. 9.6), but react intensely in the NADH reaction (Fig. 9.7). This is the typical feature of *disseminated neurogenic atrophy*, a feature which may be the only abnormality in the earliest stages of the disease, for example, in a biopsy taken from a muscle of normal strength and bulk. In atrophic muscles, on the other hand, the disease process is more advanced. In these muscles *small group atrophy*, i.e. groups of atrophic fibres of the same histochemical type (Fig. 9.8) is found, and *fibre-type grouping*, i.e. groups of fibres of the same histochemical type and of normal size, is also a feature. The former is evidence of continuing denervation after compensatory reinnervation. The latter represents effective compensatory reinnervation by axonal sprouting. Target fibres are uncommon in motor neuron disease but may occur in the early stages (Figs 9.7, 9.8). They may be more prominent in cases with a rapidly progressive course. In motor neuron disease the

Table 9.2 Pathological features in motor neuron disease

Denervation	Reinnervation	Other features
Small, angulated NADH-dark fibres	Fibre-type grouping (of normal-sized fibres)	Fibre hypertrophy (mainly Type 2 fibres)
Small group atrophy	Intermediate (Type 2C) fibres	Fibre splitting
Target fibres		Rare regenerating fibres

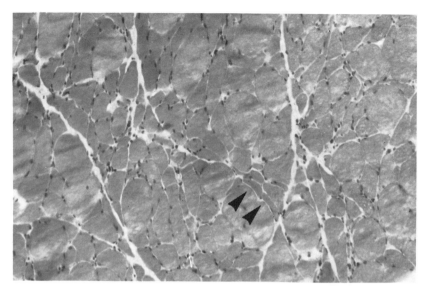

Fig. 9.5 Motor neuron disease. × 140; HE. Post-mortem specimen. There are fibres of normal size, and clusters of smaller, pointed fibres (arrows) scattered through several fascicles.

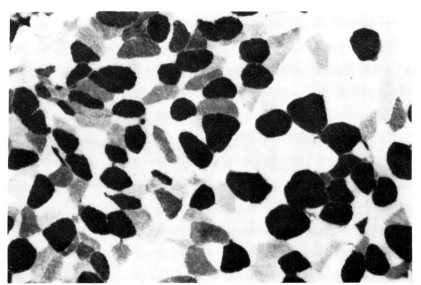

Fig. 9.6 Motor neuron disease. × 140; ATPase, pH 4.3. The biopsy consists of Type 1 (dark), Type 2C (intermediate) and Type 2A and Type 2B (pale) fibres. There are a number of atrophic pointed (denervated) fibres of either histochemical type. Fibre-type grouping is not a feature of this case.

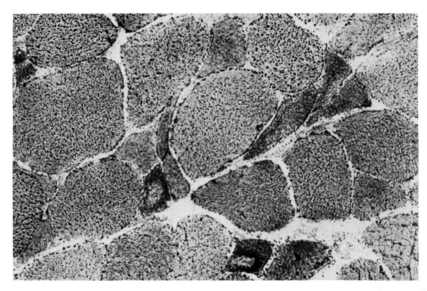

Fig. 9.7 Motor neuron disease. × 350; NADH. There are a number of pointed denervated fibres, two of which show targets. The latter are almost always restricted to Type 1 fibres.

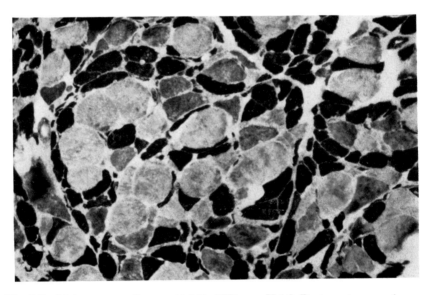

Fig. 9.8 Motor neuron disease. × 140; ATPase, pH 4.3. Post-mortem specimen. Several small groups of atrophic Type 1, and Type 2 fibres are present. Fibre-type grouping is not prominent, but there is one area of Type 1 fibre grouping at the top of the field.

groups of fibres in zones of fibre-type grouping are never as large (Fig. 9.9) as in the spinal muscular atrophies, or chronic motor neuropathies, in which whole fascicles may be of the same histochemical type. There is no inflammatory cell response in the biopsy but, rarely, focal accumulations of lymphocytes may be noted. Fibre-type grouping, especially of Type 1 fibres, has been associated with a better prognosis, and the presence of clusters of atrophic fibres (Fig. 9.10) with a poor prognosis (Patten *et al.*, 1979), reflecting the relative preponderance of compensatory reinnervation by axonal sprouting. Axonal sprouting has been directly demonstrated (Cöers *et al.*, 1973; Wohlfart, 1957) by silver impregnation and by supravital methylene blue techniques, but such methods are of limited value in diagnosis. The peripheral nerves, like the ventral roots, show Wallerian degeneration and loss of motor axons.

In patients with a more slowly progressive course the muscle biopsy may show various additional abnormalities consistent with secondary myopathic change. Indeed Achari and Anderson (1974) found changes of this type in 67% of a large series of cases. Fibre hypertrophy, mainly of Type 2 fibres (Fig. 9.11), is usually the most prominent such change, but this is not as marked as in more chronic neurogenic disorders, e.g. Type 3 spinal muscular atrophy. Fibre splitting, usually affecting these

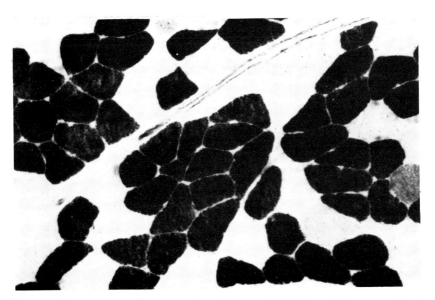

Fig. 9.9 Motor neuron disease. × 350; ATPase, pH 4.3. Type 1 fibre grouping is present, consisting of small groups (12–15 fibres), indicating that some collateral reinnervation has occurred.

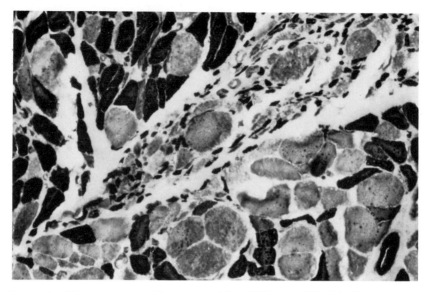

Fig. 9.10 Motor neuron disease. × 140; ATPase, pH 9.5. Post-mortem specimen. One fascicle consists of almost uniformly atrophic pointed fibres. Since these fibres do not show fibre-type grouping, they demonstrate failure of effective reinnervation. Note the difference between this appearance and that of Type 2 spinal muscular atrophy shown in Fig. 9.2.

hypertrophied fibres, may also occur and, less commonly, isolated small basophilic regenerating fibres and slight endomysial fibrosis may occur. The blood CK is sometimes slightly raised in patients with these abnormalities (Schwartz *et al.*, 1976).

In the final stages of the disease there is usually very advanced muscular wasting. Biopsies made at this time, or autopsy studies, show widespread grouped denervation atrophy, often with only a few zones of fibres of approximately normal size. Fibrosis may be prominent in the interfascicular planes. The muscle spindles are denervated and appear enlarged (Fig. 9.11), although their intrafusal muscle fibres are atrophic (Swash and Fox, 1974).

The changes in the spinal cord and brain have been reviewed by Brownell *et al.* (1970). There is atrophy of the ventral spinal roots, loss of anterior horn cells and of motor neurons in the bulbar nuclei, but sparing of the Onuf sacral nucleus that controls the striated pelvic sphincters and of the oculomotor nuclei. Some remaining motor neurons show chromatolysis and a number of different cytoplasmic intraneuronal inclusions have been noted in these cells. Bunina bodies, consisting of

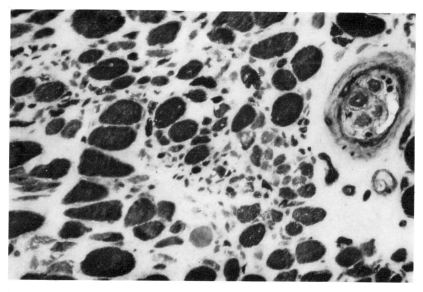

Fig. 9.11 Motor neuron disease. × 140; ATPase, pH 9.5. Post-mortem specimen. There is extensive fibre atrophy, with hypertrophy of many of the remaining functional Type 2 (dark) fibres. There are features of early secondary myopathic change consisting of rounding and increased variability in size of these Type 2 fibres. The muscle spindle appears prominent because of the loss of extrafusal skeletal muscle fibres.

eosinophilic cytoplasmic rod-like inclusions (Hirano *et al.*, 1984), and ubiquitinated filamentous inclusions are the most characteristic (Leigh *et al.*, 1988). Spheroidal axonal enlargements are frequent in the anterior horn grey matter. In addition, there is degeneration of the crossed and uncrossed corticospinal tracts, and some pallor of the spinocerebellar pathways (Swash *et al.*, 1988).

9.3   Other disorders of anterior horn cells and ventral roots

In poliomyelitis and syringomyelia the abnormalities in the muscle biopsy differ from those found in motor neuron disease. The natural history of these disorders differs from that of motor neuron disease; in poliomyelitis the disorder is not progressive, so that compensatory reinnervation is well developed and fibre-type grouping prominent (Fig. 9.12). Furthermore, secondary myopathic changes may be very marked, even to the extent that a limited histological examination, for example, using only an HE preparation, may lead to a mistaken impression of an

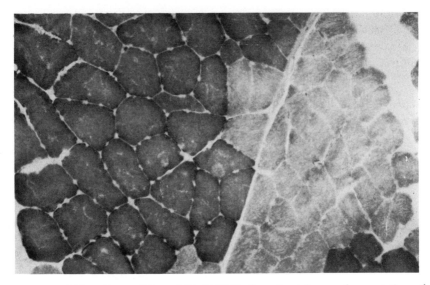

Fig. 9.12 Old poliomyelitis. × 140; NADH. Two fascicles, each consisting of Type 1 or Type 2 fibre grouping. These groups are large, indicating effective collateral reinnervation. Note that the fibres are of uniform size.

underlying myopathy (Drachman *et al.*, 1967). Lesions of the ventral (motor) roots may also cause denervation and if recovery does not occur quickly there may be features of chronic partial denervation, i.e. grouped atrophy and fibre-type grouping, in a muscle biopsy (Fig. 9.13). Denervation changes also occur in Creutzfeld–Jakob disease and in patients with viral myelitis, especially that due to *Herpes zoster*.

9.4   Polyneuropathies

Muscle biopsies are rarely of diagnostic value in polyneuropathies since the diagnosis can usually be established by the clinical features, and by electromyographic tests, including nerve conduction studies. However, in some patients with slowly progressive motor neuropathies, without sensory involvement, diagnosis may be difficult and muscle biopsy may then be useful in that it will demonstrate the neurogenic disorder and indicate its chronicity and slow rate of progression. In acute neuropathies, e.g. Guillain–Barré polyradiculoneuropathy, muscle biopsy is not an investigation of choice but, again, it may be resorted to by the clinician when there is doubt about the diagnosis, usually in order to exclude acute polymyositis. In addition, muscle biopsies are occasionally carried out for similar reasons in patients with diabetic neuropathy and

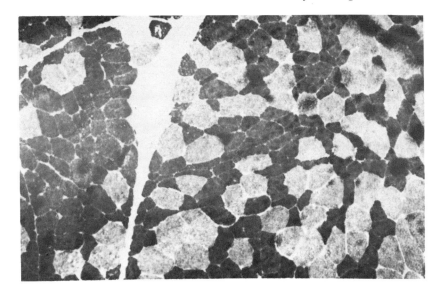

Fig. 9.13 Cervical root lesion. × 140; ATPase, pH 9.5. There is fibre-type grouping of Type 2 fibres (dark) to the left of the field. To the right there is Type 2 fibre atrophy with smaller groups of Type 2 fibres. The Type 1 fibres are of normal size and distribution.

other acute or subacute neuropathies (see Table 1.1). Small nerve fascicles in muscle biopsies may be informative in the diagnosis of certain lipid storage disorders, and in amyloid polyneuropathy, but special stains are necessary to detect the abnormality. In addition muscle biopsy may be useful in the diagnosis of mononeuropathy or polyneuropathy associated with polyarteritis nodosa or mixed connective tissue disease; about 30% of such biopsies reveal inflammation or vasculitis.

9.4.1 Chronic peripheral neuropathy

The majority of the chronic peripheral neuropathies, with prominent motor involvement, are of genetic origin (see Swash and Schwartz, 1988). The most common of these are the Types I and II forms of peroneal muscular atrophy (Charcot–Marie–Tooth disease; hereditary motor and sensory neuropathy). In the Type I disease the underlying cause is a demyelinating neuropathy in which the peripheral nerves are thickened due to reduplication of Schwannian cytoplasmic rings surrounding axons, the characteristic 'onion bulb' formations, with endoneurial fibrosis. In the Type II form the underlying abnormality is an axonal neuropathy, perhaps due to primary disease of the neuron itself. The nerve conduction velocity is very slowed in the Type I disorder, and the spinal fluid protein raised. In the Type II form, however, the nerve conduction velocity is only slightly slowed and the CSF protein is normal, or only slightly raised. The clinical features of the other forms of genetic neuropathy have been reviewed elsewhere (Dyck *et al.*, 1975; Swash and Schwartz, 1988).

(a) *Muscle biopsy.* In weak, wasted distal muscles the typical features of denervation and reinnervation are seen. These include small, angulated, atrophic fibres, which may occur in clusters, with small groups of atrophic fibres of the same histochemical type. This is associated with large groups of fibres, of one histochemical type, often comprising a whole fascicle. Individual fibres within these large groups often vary in size. Hypertrophy of Type 1 fibres is prominent, and these fibres may measure more than 150 μm in diameter. Central nucleation and fibre splitting are commonly found in such fibres and a few scattered basophilic regenerating fibres may be noted. The Type 2 fibres are often somewhat atrophic, in contrast to the Type 1 fibres, but these are also arranged in groups; fibre-type grouping is thus a feature both of Type 1 and Type 2 fibres. Target and targetoid fibres may occur. The myopathic features noted above are frequently very prominent and it is therefore essential to study biopsies of such patients with a suitable range of enzyme histochemical methods, since fibre-type grouping can only be recognized with these methods, and the diagnosis depends on this observation.

The muscle biopsy is similar in the Type I and Type II forms of the disease, despite the apparently differing underlying abnormality in the peripheral nervous system. Presumably, this indicates that axonal damage is a feature of both forms of Charcot–Marie–Tooth disease (Buchthal and Behse, 1977), although the primary abnormality in the Type I disorder affects the Schwann cells, rather than the axons. In the other genetically determined (see Table 1.1) chronic neuropathies, similar changes occur in the muscle, depending on the severity, rate of progression and duration of the motor component of the disorder. Muscle biopsies are rarely carried out in these disorders, but nerve biopsies may be useful in characterizing them, e.g. in amyloid neuropathy, leprosy and sulphatide lipidosis (metachromatic leuco-dystrophy).

9.4.2   *Acute and subacute peripheral neuropathies*

These disorders are principally characterized by denervation. Re-innervation is not prominent since the disorder is of recent onset, or acute and self-limited as in Guillain–Barré syndrome.

Table 9.3 Histological features of neurogenic disorders

	Spinal muscular atrophy		Motor neuron disease		Neuropathies	
	Types I and II	*Types III and IV*	*Early*	*Late*	*Acute*	*Chronic*
Fibre size	Small round fibres Hypertrophied fibres (Type 1)	Small angular fibres Few small rounded fibres Prominent very hypertrophied fibres (Type 1)	Scattered small angular fibres	Small and large fibres	Scattered small angular fibres or normal	Small and large fibres
Small group atrophy		+	±	+		±
Large group atrophy		+		+		+
Fibre-type grouping	+	++		+		++
Myopathic features		++		+		++

(a) *Muscle biopsy.* The hallmark of these disorders is disseminated neurogenic atrophy with little or no grouped atrophy or fibre-type grouping. Small groups of atrophic fibres may be seen scattered in the biopsy. Both fibre types show atrophy. Hypertrophy is rare. Targets and targetoid fibres may be prominent, and atrophic, angulated fibres often show prominent pyknotic nuclei. The biopsy shows no more specific features and is of little value in characterizing the cause of the neuropathy.

In *diabetic amyotrophy* similar findings occur in the early stages. Tubular aggregates may be a feature of some cases (Chokroverty *et al.*, 1977). Later in the disease, fibre-type grouping may develop. In *uraemic neuropathy*, which is reversible with effective treatment, the muscle biopsy shows little or no abnormality.

9.5   Mononeuropathies

Most mononeuropathies are due to nerve entrapment or external trauma to a nerve, and muscle biopsy is not indicated. However, in mononeuropathies associated with collagen vascular disease, e.g. poly-arteritis nodosa and other forms of autoimmune or allergic vasculitis, such as Churg–Strauss syndrome, muscle biopsy is sometimes suggested as a useful investigation. Nonetheless, random biopsy of a proximal muscle almost invariably fails to substantiate the diagnosis in patients with polyarteritis, and muscle biopsy is probably not, therefore, worth attempting in such cases (Wallace *et al.*, 1958). If muscle biopsy is arranged in an attempt to establish a diagnosis of vasculitis, a large open biopsy should be taken and transverse sections taken at multiple levels in order to search for perivascular lymphocytic, plasma cell or eosinophil infiltrates, or fibrinoid necrosis. Formalin-fixed, paraffin-embedded tissue is more convenient for this purpose than frozen tissue, perhaps the only indication for this preparative technique remaining in muscle biopsy work. Rarely, features of inflammatory myopathy and intrafascicular muscle infarction may be recognized in this disorder.

9.5.1   *Comparative features of muscle pathology in neurogenic disorders*

The various features of the major neurogenic disorders are summarized in Table 9.3.

References

Achari, A.N. and Anderson, M.S. (1974) Myopathic changes in amyotrophic lateral sclerosis. *Neurology*, **24**, 477–481.

Brownell, B., Oppenheimer, D.R. and Hughes, J.T. (1970) The central nervous system in motor neuron disease. *J. Neurol. Neurosurg. Psychiatry*, **33**, 338–357.

Buchthal, F. and Behse, F. (1977) Peroneal muscular atrophy (PMA) and related disorders. 1. Clinical manifestation as related to biopsy findings, nerve conduction and electromyography. *Brain*, **100**, 41–46.

Chokroverty, S., Reyes, M.G., Rubino, F.A. and Tonaki, H. (1977) The syndrome of diabetic amyotrophy. *Ann. Neurol.*, **2**, 181–194.

Coers, C., Telerman-Toppet, N. and Gerard, J.-M. (1973) Terminal innervation ratio in neuromuscular disease: disorders of lower motor neuron, peripheral nerve and muscle. *Arch. Neurol.*, **29**, 215–222.

DeLisle, M.B. and Carpenter, S. (1984) Neurofibrillary axonal swellings and amyotrophic lateral sclerosis. *J. Neurol. Sci.*, **63**, 241–250.

Drachman, D.B., Murphy, J.R.N., Nigam, M.P. and Hills, J.R. (1967) 'Myopathic' changes in chronically denervated muscle. *Arch. Neurol.*, **16**, 14–24.

Dubowitz, V. (1978) *Muscle Disorders in Childhood*, W.B. Saunders, London.

Dubowitz, V. and Brooke, M.H. (1973) *Muscle Biopsy – A Modern Approach*, W.B. Saunders, London.

Dyck, P.J., Thomas, P.K. and Lambert, E.M. (1975) *Peripheral Neuropathy*, Vols 1 and 2, Saunders, Philadelphia.

Hausmanowa-Petrusiewicz, I., Fidzianska, A., Niebros-Dobrosz, I. and Strugalska, M.H. (1980) Is Kugelberg–Welander spinal muscular atrophy a fetal defect? *Muscle Nerve*, **3**, 389–402.

Hirano, A., Donnenfeld, H., Sasaki, S. *et al.* (1984) The fine structure of motor neuron disease. In *Research Progress in Motor Neurone Disease* (ed. F.C. Rose), Pitman, London, pp. 328–348.

Leigh, P.N., Anderton, B.H., Dodson, A. *et al.* (1988) Ubiquitin deposits in motor neuron disease. *Neurosci. Lett.*, **93**, 197–203.

Marshall, A. and Duchen, L.W. (1975) Sensory system involvement in infantile spinal muscular atrophy. *J. Neurol. Sci.*, **26**, 349–351.

Patten, B.M., Zito, G. and Horati, Y. (1979) Histologic findings in motor neuron disease. *Arch. Neurol.*, **36**, 560–564.

Schwartz, M.S., Sargeant, M.K. and Swash, M. (1976) Longitudinal fibre splitting in neurogenic muscular disorders – its relation to the pathogenesis of myopathic change. *Brain*, **99**, 617–636.

Swash, M. and Fox, K.P. (1974) The pathology of the human muscle spindle: effect of denervation. *J. Neurol. Sci.*, **22**, 1–24.

Swash, M. and Schwartz, M.S. (1977) Implications of longitudinal muscle fibre splitting in neurogenic and myopathic disorders. *J. Neurol. Neurosurg. Psychiatry*, **40**, 1152–1159.

Swash, M. and Schwartz, M.S. (1988) *Neuromuscular Diseases: A Practical Approach to Diagnosis and Management*, 2nd edn, Springer-Verlag, Berlin, Heidelberg, New York.

Swash, M., Scholtz, C.L., Vowles, G. and Ingram, D.A. (1988) Selective and asymmetric vulnerability of corticospinal and spinocerebellar tracts in motor neuron disease. *J. Neurol. Neurosurg. Psychiatry*, **51**, 785–789.

Tomlinson, B.E., Walton, J.N. and Irving, D. (1974) Spinal cord limb motor neurons in muscular dystrophy. *J. Neurol. Sci.*, **22**, 305–327.

Wallace, S.L., Lattis, R. and Ragan, C. (1958) Diagnostic significance of the muscle biopsy. *Am. J. Med.*, **25**, 600–610.

Weller, R.O., Swash, M., McLellan, D.L. and Scholtz, C. (1983) *Clinical Neuropathology*, Springer-Verlag, Heidelberg, Berlin, New York.

Wohlfart, G. (1957) Collateral regeneration from residual motor nerve fibres in amyotrophic lateral sclerosis. *Neurology*, **7**, 124–134.

10 Tumours of striated muscle and related disorders

In collaboration with Jon van der Walt

Tumours presenting in striated muscle are uncommon. Most are primary tumours but few of these in fact represent primary tumours of muscle cells since neoplasms arising in other tissues within muscle, for example fibrous tissue, blood vessels, fat and nerve fibres, are more common. In addition, neoplasms arising in contiguous structures such as bone or cartilage, may invade muscle. Metastases in muscle are rarely clinically apparent, and thus unlikely to present for biopsy (Doshi and Fowler, 1983). However, microscopic metastases are more common, occurring in 16% of one series of patients with malignant disease studied at autopsy (Pearson, 1959). CT imaging is useful in the clinical assessment of soft-tissue tumours, and in the detection of metastases (Golding and Husband, 1982).

Metastatic tumours in muscle are more commonly lymphomas than carcinomas. Primary lymphomas may also rarely arise in muscle (Lanham *et al.*, 1989). Tumour spread to muscle by cancer from other sites most frequently occurs by extension of the tumour from neighbouring structures. Tumour invasion occurs along fascial planes or even along the sarcolemmal tubes of the muscle fibres themselves (Slatkin and Pearson, 1976). The muscle may be further damaged by the effects of compression by the tumour on the muscle, on its nerve supply, or on its blood vessels, causing infarction, haemorrhage, oedema and thus regenerative changes, or features of denervation in the muscle at the margins of the tumour.

10.1 Primary tumours arising in muscle

A classification of primary tumours arising in muscle is given in Table 10.1. Many of these lesions are uncommon in limb muscles. Other mass lesions, sometimes referred to as pseudotumours, consisting of proliferative or inflammatory changes, may also present as muscle tumours (Table 10.2).

There are no reliable physical signs to distinguish between a reactive, benign or malignant soft-tissue mass (Enzinger and Weiss, 1988). Biopsy

Table 10.1   Commoner primary tumours arising in muscle

Tumours of muscle tissue
  Benign
    rhabdomyoma
    leiomyoma
  Malignant
    rhabdomyosarcoma
      embryonal
      alveolar
      pleomorphic
    leiomyosarcoma

Tumours of fibrous tissue
  Fibromatosis
    superficial (fascial) fibromatoses
    deep (musculoaponeurotic) fibromatoses
  Malignant
    fibrosarcoma

Fibrohistiocytic tumours
  Malignant
    malignant fibrous histiocytoma

Tumours of fat
  Benign
    intramuscular lipoma
    hibernoma
  Malignant
    liposarcoma

Tumours of blood vessels
  Benign
    intramuscular haemangioma
    haemangiopericytoma
  Malignant
    epithelioid haemangioendothelioma
    angiosarcoma

Tumours of peripheral nerve
  Benign
    neurilemmoma and neurofibroma
    granular-cell tumour
  Malignant
    malignant schwannoma

Other tumours that may arise in muscle
  Benign
    intramuscular myxoma
  Malignant
    synovial sarcoma
    alveolar soft-part sarcoma
    clear-cell sarcoma
    epithelioid sarcoma
    extraskeletal chondrosarcoma
    extraskeletal osteosarcoma
    malignant lymphoma

Table 10.2   Masses that mimic tumours (pseudotumours)

Haematoma

Reactive and inflammatory lesions
   Intramuscular nodular fasciitis
   Proliferative myositis
   Focal myositis
   Myositis ossificans

Infections
   Parasites
   Fungi

is therefore required in most cases. Needle biopsy does not play a major role in the diagnosis of soft-tissue masses. Sampling error may lead the pathologist to an incorrect diagnosis or underestimation of the grade of a sarcoma. To avoid contamination of the wound, excisional biopsies should be confined to lesions smaller than 3 cm in size. Incisional biopsies should be used for larger lesions and the site carefully chosen to allow definitive surgical excision if required. Frozen section is less reliable than paraffin sections. At all times, close consultation between surgeon and pathologist is mandatory.

10.2   Tumours of muscle

10.2.1   Benign tumours

Extracardiac rhabdomyoma is a rare benign lesion of striated muscle. Controversy exists as to whether it is a benign neoplasm or a hamartoma (Enzinger and Weiss, 1988). Most examples are solitary but rarely they may be multifocal (Blaauwgeers *et al.*, 1989). It predominantly affects men older than 40 years and is almost invariably found in the head and neck region. The tumour consists of large polygonal cells, frequently containing vacuoles staining positively with PAS for glycogen on frozen section. The cells (Fig. 10.1) show cross-striations and unique 'jackstraw' crystalline inclusions which are enhanced in the PTAH stain. The cells stain positively for desmin and myoglobin. Electron microscopy reveals well-formed filaments with Z-bands. Mitoses are rare. Local excision usually effects permanent cure (Enzinger and Weiss, 1988).

  Leiomyoma of the deep soft tissues is rare and may occur in the extremities, abdominal cavity, or retroperitoneum (Enzinger and Weiss, 1988). The tumours arise from smooth muscle cells, and origin from vessel walls may be demonstrable. Many undergo degenerative changes

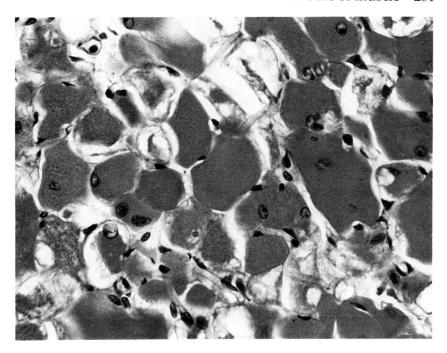

Fig. 10.1 Rhabdomyoma. × 493; HE. The biopsy consists of vacuolated polygonal cells with vesicular nuclei, resembling myoblasts. Many cells show cross-striations.

and become calcified. The distinction from leiomyosarcoma may be difficult, but true leiomyomas are benign.

10.2.2 Malignant tumours

Rhabdomyosarcoma represents 10–20% of all sarcomas of soft-tissue origin, and is the most common soft-tissue sarcoma of childhood. Three histological types are recognized. Embryonal rhabdomyosarcoma is commonest in children under 10 years of age. Botryoid features, i.e. an appearance resembling bunches of grapes, occur in this type. The alveolar type is less common, accounting for 10–20% of tumours (Enzinger and Weiss, 1988), and occurs in young adults (Enzinger and Shiraki, 1969). The pleomorphic type is the least common and has its peak incidence after 45 years of age (Enzinger and Weiss, 1988). Embryonal rhabdomyosarcomas usually arise in the orbit, nasopharynx, lower urogenital tract and bile duct. The alveolar type has a similar distribution but has a much higher incidence in the upper and lower extremities. The pleomorphic variants arise in the limb muscles, and to a lesser extent in the trunk. The thigh is the commonest site of origin of pleomorphic rhabdomyosarcomas but alveolar tumours arise with equal frequency in arms, legs and trunk muscles.

Microscopically, embryonal rhabdomyosarcoma (Fig. 10.2) is composed of a variety of different types of tumour cells, with varying patterns of cellular organization so that cellular, round or spindle cell areas may alternate with myxoid areas in the same tumour. Fibrosed areas may be a feature and areas of immature bone or cartilage may be found. The predominant cell type is the embryonal rhabdomyoblast. When undifferentiated this is a small, round to oval cell with a prominent vesicular nucleus. Larger cells, which may show cross-striations on HE and PTAH staining, are found in more differentiated areas of the tumour. Myofibrils can more easily be identified in ATPase and NADH preparations of frozen material (Sarnat *et al.*, 1979). In the botryoid variant the cells lie in a myxoid stroma sometimes with a zone of submucosal cellularity termed

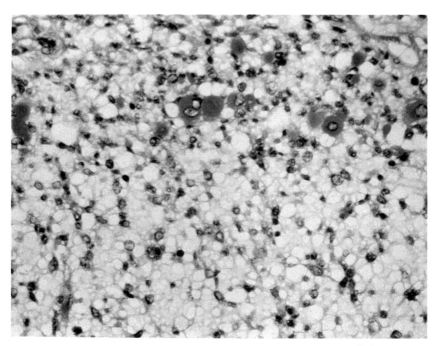

Fig. 10.2 Embryonal rhabdomyosarcoma. × 123; HE. The cellular pattern shows round and spindle cells, mixed with myxoid areas. The cells are of relatively uniform size, and their cytoplasm and nuclei are thinly stained. Some isolated larger cells are present.

the 'cambium layer'. The alveolar rhabdomyosarcoma (Fig. 10.3) shows a characteristic alveolar pattern but may also contain solid cellular areas. Multinucleated giant cells are common (Enzinger and Weiss, 1988). Mitoses are found in all three types but are commonest in the embryonal form. Bizarre, multinucleated cells, vacuolated cells and cells containing large nucleoli are frequently found in the uncommon pleomorphic type, which must be distinguished from other pleomorphic sarcomas such as malignant fibrous histiocytoma and pleomorphic liposarcoma that are much more common.

Ultrastructural studies reveal myofibrils but few cytoplasmic organelles, the appearances resembling those of myoblasts. The more differentiated cells react with antibodies to desmin, the predominant intermediate filament in muscle, and myoglobin but less well-differentiated cells react less strongly with myoglobin. Desmin is therefore the preferred marker for diagnosis of these tumours (Garger *et al.*, 1981; Dodd *et al.*, 1989). Myosin and actin markers are less useful. Rhabdomyoblastic differentiation may be found in other tumours such as malignant schwannoma, malignant mesenchymoma, Wilms' tumour,

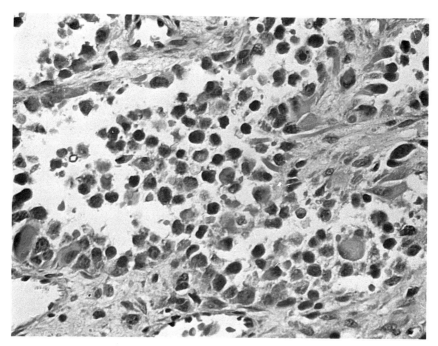

Fig. 10.3 Alveolar rhabdomyoma. × 317; HE. The tumour shows an alveolar pattern, with more solid areas; some cells are multinucleated.

carcinosarcoma, chondrosarcoma, malignant mixed Müllerian tumour of the uterus and various germ-cell tumours amongst others, and it must always be considered in context. Rhabdomyosarcomas metastasize widely through the blood stream, and the metastases resemble the primary neoplasm. Survival has improved markedly with multi-disciplinary therapeutic regimes, and with localized tumours it is greater than 70% at 5 years. However, distant spread at time of presentation confers a poor prognosis, only 20% of patients with metastatic disease at time of presentation surviving 5 years.

Leiomyosarcoma in contrast to its benign counterpart, has a predeliction for deep sites of origin (Enzinger and Weiss, 1988), and is an uncommon primary tumour in muscle. It is composed of interlacing bands of spindle cells with variable degrees of pleomorphism (Fig. 10.4). Epithelioid, myxoid and granular variants are described. In well-differentiated examples, malignancy is chiefly determined by the mitotic count. However it is never possible to be certain that a smooth-muscle tumour is benign, particularly if it is large (Enzinger and Weiss, 1988).

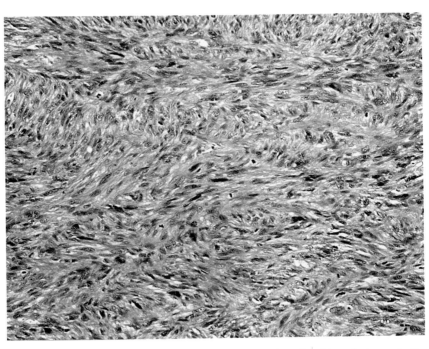

Fig. 10.4 Leiomyosarcoma. × 123; HE. There are bands of interlacing spindle cells, with some pleomorphic areas.

10.3   Tumours of fibrous tissue

These are classified as fibromatoses and malignant fibrosarcomas (Table 10.1). The latter are uncommon.

10.3.1   Fibromatoses

The fibromatoses consist of a group of infiltrating fibroblastic pro-liferations of similar appearance which infiltrate surrounding tissues, tend to recur locally, but never metastasize. Reactive and inflammatory conditions are excluded. The fibromatoses may be divided into superficial and deep types (Enzinger and Weiss, 1988). Superficial fibromatoses are small, slow-growing lesions that rarely involve deeper structures. The commonest site of origin is the palm of the hand (Dupuytren's contracture). Plantar, penile and knuckle-pad fibromatoses are less common. Microscopically they show an initial cellular, proliferative appearance which progresses to a late collagenous phase.

Deep or musculoaponeurotic fibromatoses (desmoid tumours) grow rapidly, infiltrate surrounding tissues, and may become large. The peak age incidence is between 10 and 40 years of age. They may occur in abdominal, intra-abdominal and extra-abdominal sites (Table 10.3). Extra-abdominal fibromatoses occur at a wide range of sites but the shoulder, followed by chest wall and back, thigh and mesentery are the commonest sites (Enzinger and Weiss, 1988). Microscopically, they are composed of interlacing bundles of fibroblasts in a collagenous stroma. Mitoses are scarce. Occasionally this cellularity may lead to confusion with fibrosarcomas or reactive proliferations such as nodular fasciitis. There is a marked tendency to local recurrence but it is not possible to predict the behaviour of the tumour from the microscopic appearances. The recurrence rate depends largely on the completeness of local excision (Enzinger and Weiss, 1988).

Table 10.3   The fibromatoses (after Enzinger and Weiss, 1988)

Superficial (fascial) fibromatoses
   Palmar fibromatosis (Dupuytren's contracture)
   Plantar fibromatosis (Ledderhose's disease)
   Penile fibromatosis (Peyronie's disease)
   Knuckle-pads

Deep (musculoaponeurotic) fibromatoses
   Extra-abdominal fibromatosis (extra-abdominal desmoid)
   Abdominal fibromatosis (abdominal desmoid)
   Intra-abdominal fibromatosis (intra-abdominal desmoid)
      (pelvic fibromatosis)

Fibromatoses in infancy and childhood show similar behaviour to the adult forms. Infantile digital, gingival, hyaline and desmoid type fibromatoses and calcifying aponeurotic fibroma tend to recur locally but fibromatosis colli, fibrous hamartoma of infancy and infantile myofibromatosis rarely recur (Enzinger and Weiss, 1988).

10.3.2   Fibrosarcoma

Many tumours that were once diagnosed as fibrosarcomas are now classified as fibromatoses, malignant fibrous histiocytoma, malignant schwannoma, synovial sarcoma and other entities, making this an uncommon diagnosis in modern practice.

Fibrosarcoma occurs most commonly in the thigh musculature as a firm, circumscribed mass. The mean age of onset is the fifth decade and the duration of survival is related to the location and histological grade of malignancy; deeply seated and highly cellular tumours having the worst prognosis. Metastases occur through the blood stream to lung, liver and bone in about 60% of cases. About 50% of cases survive five years from diagnosis (Pritchard et al., 1974). Five year survival is improved from only 30% after local excision to 80% after radical excision (Bizer, 1971).

The tumour is of variable histological type. Some tumours consist of a large amount of collagen, containing fibroblasts of varying size and shape in interlaced bands often arranged in a herringbone pattern. In others there is less collagen, the tumour is more cellular, and the cells are spindle-shaped without evidence of differentiation. Mitotic figures are frequent. There may be difficulty in distinguishing this tumour from malignant fibrous histiocytoma, monophasic synovial sarcoma, malignant schwannoma and even spindle-cell carcinoma. Negative immunoperoxidase staining for cytokeratin and S-100 protein lends support to the diagnosis.

10.4   Fibrohistiocytic tumours

Benign fibrous histiocytomas occur in superficial sites and do not involve muscle.

Malignant fibrous histiocytoma is the commonest sarcoma of late adult life (Enzinger and Weiss, 1988). Storiform, pleomorphic, myxoid, giant-cell, inflammatory and angiomatoid subtypes have been described. The angiomatoid subtype occurs in the dermis and subcutis and does not involve muscle. The other subtypes commonly involve skeletal muscle of the extremities and may be considered together (Enzinger and Weiss, 1988).

Malignant fibrous histiocytomas are rare in children and two-thirds

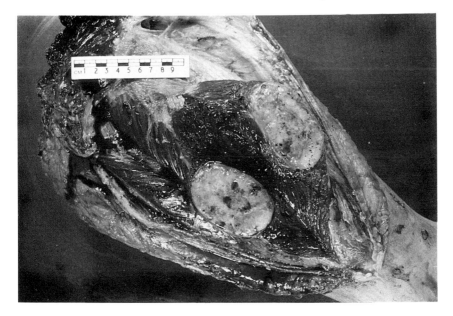

Fig. 10.5 Amputation of thigh. The rounded tumour was a malignant fibrous histiocytoma, arising in the muscles of the posterior thigh.

occur in adult males. The lower limbs are affected most commonly (Fig. 10.5), followed by the upper limbs and retroperitoneal tissue (Enzinger and Weiss, 1988). Fever and leucocytosis have been noted, particularly with the inflammatory subtype and hypoglycaemia may rarely occur (Enzinger and Weiss, 1988). The tumour may follow irradiation but no other aetiological factors are established (Weiss and Enzinger, 1978). Metastases occur in up to 50% of cases (Weiss, 1982). The tumours usually present as multilobulated, fleshy masses up to 10 cm in diameter. The inflammatory subtype may appear yellow, due to accumulated lipid; the myxoid form is soft and translucent.

The microscopic appearances are variable, ranging from a storiform pattern to a highly pleomorphic tumour (Fig. 10.6). Myxoid (Fig. 10.7), inflammatory (Fig. 10.8) and xanthomatous change may be superadded. Electron microscopy and immunohistochemistry yield conflicting results (Hirose *et al.*, 1989), but may be useful in excluding other lesions. The origin of malignant fibrous histiocytoma is controversial. Recent immunohistochemical studies (Lawson *et al.*, 1987) support the concept that malignant fibrous histiocytoma is a tumour of mesenchymal cells with the propensity to differentiate in several different directions, rather than a tumour of monocyte/macrophage lineage.

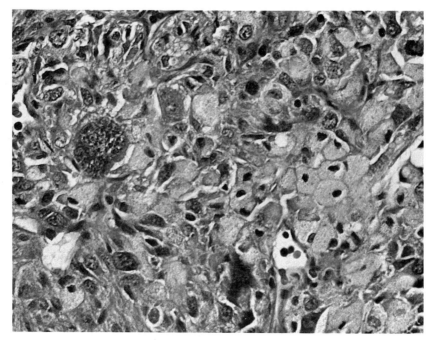

Fig. 10.6 Malignant fibrous histiocytoma. × 493; HE. The tumour has a pleomorphic cellular appearance, with giant cells, vacuolated cells, and marked variation in nuclear morphology.

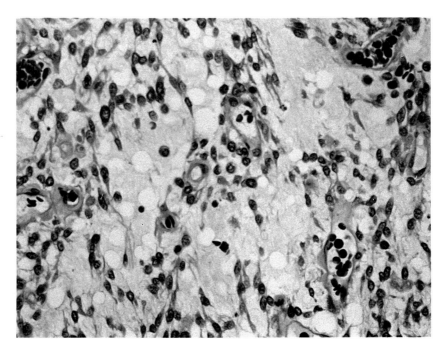

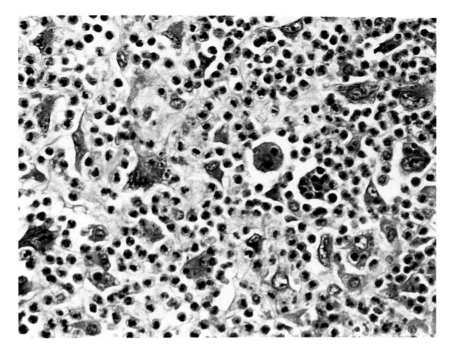

Fig. 10.8   Malignant fibrous histiocytoma. × 493; HE. The tumour shows large, multinucleated malignant cells, interspersed with inflammatory cells, and with some myxoid change.

10.5   Tumours of fat

10.5.1   Benign tumours

Intramuscular lipomas are common. As a rule the fat cells in the lipoma are well differentiated (Fig. 10.9) and this serves to distinguish this benign tumour from liposarcoma. However, an atypical appearance has been described in intramuscular lipomas (Evans *et al.*, 1979).

   Hibernoma is a rare tumour of brown fat consisting of granular or vacuolated acidophilic cells. The tumour usually presents in the shoulder or neck and may involve muscle.

Fig. 10.7   Malignant fibrous histiocytoma. × 493; HE. There is a myxoid appearance to this tumour, separating areas of more marked cellularity.

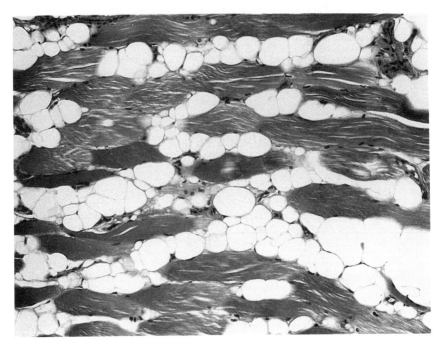

Fig. 10.9   Benign intramuscular lipoma. × 308; HE. The tumour consists of areas of fatty infiltration of the striated muscular tissue.

10.5.2   *Malignant tumours*

Liposarcoma (Fig. 10.10) is the second most common sarcoma after malignant fibrous histiocytoma (Enzinger and Weiss, 1988). The commonest sites are the thigh and retroperitoneal tissues, where the tumours may attain huge size. The median age of presentation is in the sixth decade and liposarcomas in childhood are rare (Enzinger and Weiss, 1988). The myxoid type is the commonest and consists of lipoblasts in varying stages of development in a myxoid matrix with a characteristic 'chicken wire' vascular pattern. The round-cell type often shows transition to the myxoid form. The well-differentiated type resembles a lipoma but variable numbers of lipoblasts are found. Pleomorphic liposarcoma contains bizarre giant cells, which may contain fat, and is difficult to distinguish from pleomorphic malignant fibrous histiocytoma or rhabdomyosarcoma. Lipid may be demonstrated in the lipoblasts by the oil red O stain but many other sarcomas contain intracellular fat, and this is not a diagnostic appearance. Over half of all liposarcomas recur, the five-year survival rate varying from 57 to 70% (Enzinger and Weiss,

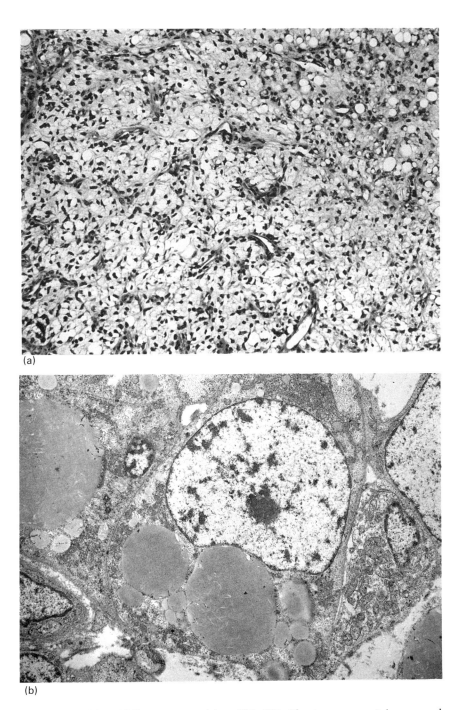

(a)

(b)

Fig. 10.10 Myxoid liposarcoma. (a) × 123; HE. The tumour contains several elements, consisting of a myxoid and vascular stroma, and vacuolated fat cells. (b) Electron micrograph showing characteristic indentation of the lipoblast nucleus by fat droplets.

1988). Superficial tumours and well-differentiated and myxoid types have a favourable prognosis, while deep tumours and those of round-cell or pleomorphic type are more aggressive.

10.6   Tumours of blood vessels

10.6.1   Benign tumours

Intramuscular haemangioma (Fig. 10.11) may be capillary, cavernous or arteriovenous. These tumours may diffusely infiltrate skeletal muscle, and are found chiefly in young adults. They are histologically and clinically benign but their pseudoinfiltrative pattern may lead to a mistaken diagnosis of malignancy (Allen and Enzinger, 1972).

10.6.2   Haemangiopericytoma

Haemangiopericytoma most commonly arises in the thigh, pelvic fossa or retroperitoneum of adults as a painless, well-circumscribed mass. The

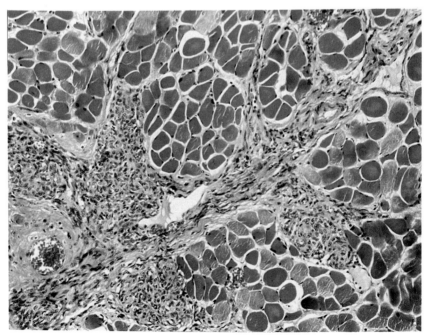

Fig. 10.11   Intramuscular haemangioma. × 123; HE. There is a prominent endothelial-cell-derived proliferation displacing and infiltrating the muscle tissue.

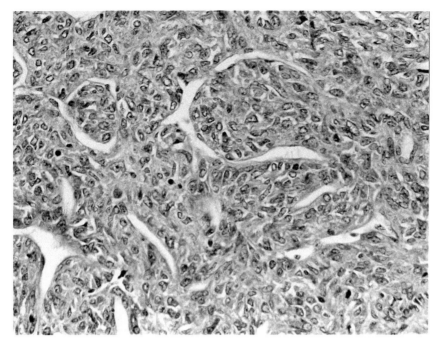

Fig. 10.12   Haemangiopericytoma. × 308; HE. The tumour consists of tightly packed, round, oval or spindle-shaped cells, arranged in a pseudoglandular pattern, with thin-walled vascular spaces.

tumour (Fig. 10.12) consists of tightly packed uniform round, oval or spindle-shaped cells surrounding thin-walled vascular spaces giving the characteristic 'antler' or 'staghorn' vessels. Factor VIII-related antigen delineates the vascular spaces very well but is not of value in diagnosis. It may be difficult to distinguish this tumour from other well-vascularized mesenchymal tumours such as synovial sarcoma and malignant fibrous histiocytoma. Haematogenous metastases occur in about 15% of cases of malignant haemangiopericytoma. The presence of mitotic figures, increased cellularity, pleomorphism and haemorrhage and necrosis are important prognostic features (Enzinger and Smith, 1976).

10.6.3   Malignant tumours

Epithelioid haemangioendothelioma pursues a clinical course intermediate between haemangioma and angiosarcoma (Weiss *et al.*, 1986). The tumour arises at any age after early childhood in superficial or deep tissues. Approximately half arise from a blood vessel. Microscopically the diagnostic hallmark is the formation of strands and nests of epithelioid cells that may contain intracytoplasmic lumina. Cytokeratins are not expressed but factor VIII-related antigen is usually found (Weiss *et al.*, 1986).

Angiosarcomas are rare tumours and only about one-quarter of the total occur in deep sites (Enzinger and Weiss, 1988). They are composed (Fig. 10.13) of vascular channels lined by neoplastic endothelial cells of varying differentiation. Solid and spindle-cell areas are found and factor VIII-related antigen is variably expressed.

10.7   Tumours of peripheral nerves

10.7.1   *Benign tumours*

Neurofibromas and neurilemmomas are closely related tumours derived from the Schwann cell of peripheral nerves. Both occur most commonly in superficial locations, but in von Recklinghausen's disease, multiple

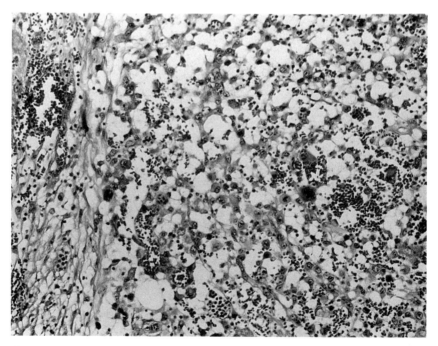

Fig. 10.13   Angiosarcoma. × 123; HE. There are prominent vascular channels and sinusoids containing erythrocytes, and lined by hypertrophic endothelial cells of varying degrees of differentiation.

neurofibromas may occur in deep sites. Both are composed of spindle cells characteristically arranged in a 'palisaded' pattern with areas of variable cellular density; the Antoni A and B patterns. Solitary lesions are benign but in von Recklinghausen's disease, malignant transformation may occur (Enzinger and Weiss, 1988).

Granular-cell schwannoma (Fig. 10.14) occurs in adult life at any site. The commonest sites are the tongue, the chest wall and the upper limbs. Most tumours are superficial. This tumour was formerly termed 'granular cell myoblastoma', but electron microscopy (Fisher and Wechsler, 1962) and immunohistochemical localization of S-100 protein (Nakazato *et al.*, 1982) have established its neural origin.

10.7.2 Malignant tumours

Malignant schwannomas account for approximately 10% of sarcomas, half of these arising in the setting of von Recklinghausen's disease (Enzinger and Weiss, 1988). The peak incidence is between 20 and 50 years of age.

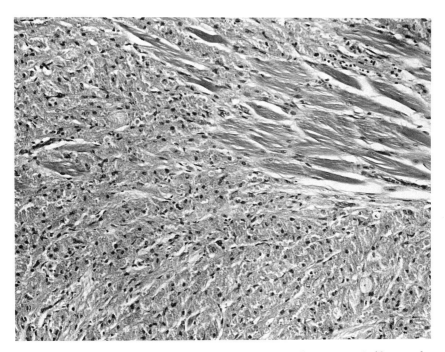

Fig. 10.14 Granular cell myoblastoma. × 123; HE. The tumour infiltrates the muscle tissue, and consists of plump or elongated cells with centrally located nuclei, many of which are enlarged or irregularly pyknotic.

Most arise from major nerve trunks, the commonest sites being the proximal parts of upper and lower limbs, and trunk (Enzinger and Weiss, 1988; Ghosh *et al.*, 1973). Referred pain, paraesthesias and weakness may accompany the development of a mass (Enzinger and Weiss, 1988).

Macroscopically, the tumours resemble other sarcomas, but a neural origin is usually demonstrable. Microscopically they resemble fibrosarcomas but Antoni A and B patterns and nuclear palisading may be seen. Positive immunostaining for S-100 protein (Fig. 10.15) occurs in up to 90% of cases (Enzinger and Weiss, 1988) and is helpful in establishing the diagnosis. In rare cases, rhabdomyoblasts may be found in an otherwise typical malignant schwannoma – the so-called Triton tumour.

Peripheral neuroepithelioma is a rare primitive neuroectodermal tumour composed of small round cells, sometimes forming rosettes. Most occur before the age of 35 years, most commonly in buttock and upper thigh (Enzinger and Weiss, 1988). Immunostaining is positive for neuron-specific enolase but negative for S-100 protein (Hashimoto *et al.*, 1983).

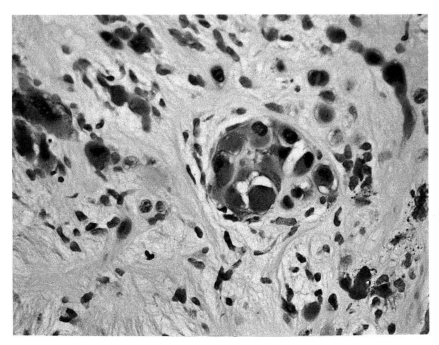

Fig. 10.15 Epithelioid malignant Schwannoma. × 493; Immunoperoxidase; S-100 protein. The cellular elements are reactive to the S-100 antibody, indicating their homology with the Schwann cells.

Extraskeletal Ewing's sarcoma is a similar or possibly identical tumour. Nearly half arise in the chest wall or paravertebral region (Enzinger and Weiss, 1988).

10.8   Other tumours that may arise in muscle

10.8.1   Benign tumours

Intramuscular myxomas are benign tumours of adult life that arise in the large muscles of the thigh, shoulder, buttock and upper arm. They may readily be recognized by the mucoid material, consisting largely of hyaluronic acid, in which small round or spindle-shaped cells, reticulin and sparse collagen fibrils can be seen. They probably derive from fibroblasts which produce excess amounts of glycosaminoglycans and must be distinguished from myxoid change in other benign and malignant soft tissue tumours (Mackenzie, 1981).

10.8.2   Malignant tumours

Alveolar soft-part sarcoma arises in a range of locations but most commonly in the extremities, one-third arising in the thigh (Lieberman *et al.*, 1966). The tumour is commoner in women, and usually presents in the third or fourth decade (Enzinger and Weiss, 1988). It infiltrates soft tissues and metastasizes widely. Microscopically, it consists of polygonal, coarsely granular cells arranged in an alveolar pattern (Fig. 10.16) or in compact groups. These cells have an eosinophilic cytoplasm which stains light brown in trichrome and PTAH stains. PAS-positive, diastase-resistant intracytoplasmic, needle-like structures with characteristic crystalline 58–100 Å periodicity at electron microscopy, are found in these cells (Fisher and Reidford, 1971). Endothelial cell-lined, thin vascular channels and septa are prominent. Mitotic figures are usually present. The tumour may be of rhabdomyoblastic origin. The tumour cells contain desmin, actin, vimentin and Z-band protein (Mukai *et al.*, 1984; Foschini *et al.*, 1988).

Synovial sarcoma presents most commonly in the region of the knee, foot and ankle joints and may occur at any age (Enzinger and Weiss, 1988). Two microscopical features are characteristic – a spindle-cell fibrosarcoma-like element and an epithelioid element. The epithelioid elements stain positively for epithelial markers in contrast to normal and hyperplastic synovium, which is negative (Miettinen and Virtanen, 1984). Synovial sarcoma is therefore probably a misnomer and 'carcinosarcoma of soft tissues' might be a more appropriate term (Miettinen and Virtanen, 1984). Well-differentiated tumours carry a better prognosis, but the five-year survival is only about 50%.

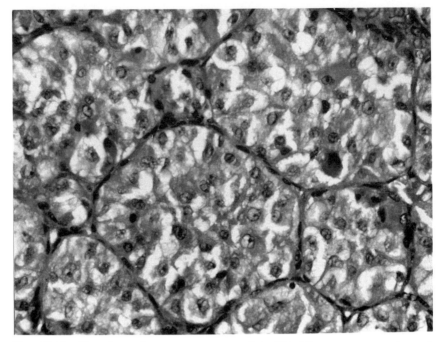

Fig. 10.16 Alveolar soft-part sarcoma. × 493; HE. The tumour consists of coarsely granular cells arranged in an alveolar pattern, with prominent, thin septa separating clusters of cells.

Malignant melanoma of soft parts is the preferred term for 'clear-cell sarcoma of tendons and aponeuroses'. Most examples occur in the second to fourth decades, predominantly in the lower extremity (Chung and Enzinger, 1983). Microscopically the tumour is composed of nests of clear and granular eosinophilic rounded fusiform cells, packeted by fibrous septa (Fig. 10.17). Melanin and S-100 protein can be demonstrated in the majority of cases and melanosomes may be detected by electron microscopy. The prognosis is poor, with frequent metastases to lung, lymph nodes and bone.

Epithelioid sarcoma mostly occurs in the second to fourth decades in the extremities, the distal arm and hand being involved in more than half the cases (Chase and Enzinger, 1985). The tumour is seldom protuberant and often presents as an infiltrating mass in the superficial or deep tissues, or as a diffuse swelling, particularly in the hand. Microscopically it is composed of a nodular growth of fusiform or plump epithelioid cells, often centrally necrotic (Fig. 10.18). The 'pseudogranulomatous' pattern may lead to confusion with reactive and inflammatory conditions. Most cases react with antibodies to cytokeratins (Chase and Enzinger, 1985). Clinically epithelioid sarcomas pursue an indolent but relentless clinical course characterized by recurrences in up to 77% and metastases in 45% of cases. Lymph nodes are the commonest site of metastases, followed by the lungs (Chase and Enzinger, 1985). The histogenesis is unknown.

Primary bone and cartilage-forming tumours presenting in muscle are rare and must be distinguished from direct extension of primary bone tumours. A range of benign and malignant bone and cartilage-forming tumours have been described (Reiman and Dahlin, 1986) which resemble those arising primarily in bone. Tumours which might have been classified as well-differentiated chondrosarcomas, had they arisen in bone, do not metastasize when they originate in the soft tissues. Thus, the criteria of cellular change required for a diagnosis of malignancy in an osseous primary tumour do not apply at extraosseous primary sites. However, extraosseous myxoid and mesenchymal chondrosarcomas and osteosarcomas have a poor prognosis (Reiman and Dahlin, 1986).

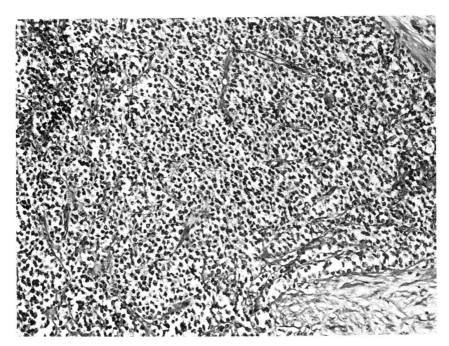

Fig. 10.17   Clear-cell sarcoma. × 123; HE. The tumour consists of clear, rounded or fusiform cells; it is sometimes termed 'malignant melanoma of soft parts' and there is doubt as to the nosological status of these two terms.

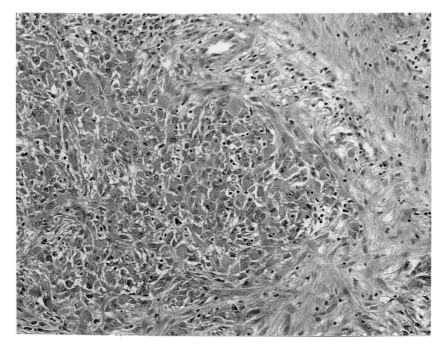

Fig. 10.18 Epithelioid sarcoma. × 123; HE. The tumour consists of a collagenous matrix, containing plump, oval or spindle-shaped cells, with some central areas of necrosis.

Malignant lymphomas may occur in muscle as an infiltrating mass, most commonly in the thigh (Lanham *et al.*, 1989). Hodgkin's disease and lymphoblastic lymphoma are not recognized in muscle, but all other histological types are represented (Lanham *et al.*, 1989). Positive staining for lymphoid markers distinguishes malignant lymphoma from other round-cell tumours.

10.9 Masses that mimic tumours (pseudotumours)

A wide range of benign and reactive conditions may present in the soft tissues and mimic sarcomas because of their rapid growth, propensity to infiltrate adjacent structures and microscopical cellularity, atypicality and mitotic activity (Ross *et al.*, 1982). It is a paradox that sarcomas frequently appear encapsulated while reactive, proliferating masses may have an infiltrative border. Some of the commoner entities affecting muscle are discussed here. Local excision is adequate in all cases and very few recur locally.

10.9.1   Reactive and inflammatory lesions

Intramuscular nodular fasciitis presents most commonly in young adults aged between 20 and 35 years of age as a rapidly growing mass, nearly half occurring on the upper extremity (Enzinger and Weiss, 1988). Microscopically the lesion consists of proliferating immature fibroblasts in a reticulin-rich stroma (Fig. 10.19) in which lymphocytes and areas of haemorrhage may be found. Mitoses are frequent and muscle fibres may be entrapped at the periphery of the lesion.

Proliferative myositis presents as a rapidly growing, poorly demarcated, scar-like, indurated mass in muscle usually occurring in a patient older than 45 years and particularly affecting muscles of the trunk. Histologically there are two main features; fibroblastic proliferation, involving the epimysium and endomysium, and large basophilic giant cells resembling ganglion cells (Enzinger and Dulcey, 1967). Proliferative fasciitis is closely related but arises more superficially (Chung and Enzinger, 1975).

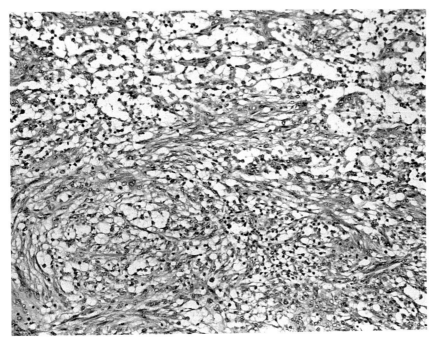

Fig. 10.19   Nodular fasciitis. × 123; HE. The biopsy consists of bundles of proliferating fibroblasts, with a lymphocytic cellular infiltration; muscle fibres may be trapped in the lesion, which is benign.

Focal myositis presents as a slowly enlarging mass within the soft tissues of an extremity, usually in adults. At surgery it appears pale and poorly demarcated from surrounding muscle. Microscopically the appearances are of necrotic muscle with inflammation, phagocytosis, regeneration and fibrosis. The cause is unknown (Heffner *et al.*, 1977).

Myositis ossificans presents as a diffuse, soft mass, which with the passage of time becomes hard and indurated. Half the cases occur in young patients aged 20–30 years and most cases occur in the muscles of the limbs (Enzinger and Weiss, 1988). Microscopically the lesion has three distinct zones of immature fibroblastic tissue centrally, surrounded by a zone of immature osteogenic tissue forming osteoid, which may develop peripherally into mature bone. This zonal arrangement is the reverse of that found in osteogenic sarcoma from which it must be distinguished (Enzinger and Weiss, 1988).

Conclusion

Although the diagnosis of tumours arising in muscle is often difficult it is particularly important to recognize those tumours whose biological behaviour is malignant, since the treatment of choice in the latter is wide surgical excision. Benign lesions simply require adequate local excision. In determining the prognosis of tumours arising in muscle, the cell of origin, degree of differentiation, and stage are important. Immuno-histochemical techniques for diagnosis, using monoclonal markers for cytoskeletal and membrane proteins, are indispensable in their precise classification (Angervall *et al.*, 1986).

References

Allen, P.W. and Enzinger, F.M. (1972) Hemangioma of skeletal muscle. An analysis of 89 cases. *Cancer*, **29**, 8–22.

Angervall, L., Kindblom, L.-G., Rydholm, A. and Stener, B. (1986) The diagnosis and prognosis of soft tissue tumours. *Semin. Diagn. Pathol.*, **3**, 240–258.

Bizer, L.S. (1971) Fibrosarcoma report of 64 cases. *Am. J. Surg.*, **121**, 586–594.

Blaauwgeers, J.L.G., Troost, D., Dingemans, K.P. *et al.* (1989) Multifocal rhabdomyoma of the neck. Report of a case studied by fine needle aspiration, light and electron microscopy, histochemistry and immunohistochemistry. *Am. J. Surg. Pathol.*, **13**, 791–799.

Chase, D.R. and Enzinger, F.M. (1985) Epithelioid sarcoma. Diagnosis, prognostic indicators and treatment. *Am. J. Surg. Pathol.*, **9**, 241–243.

Chung, E.B. and Enzinger, F.M. (1975) Proliferative fasciitis. *Cancer*, **36**, 1450–1458.

Chung, E.B. and Enzinger, F.M. (1983) Malignant melanoma of soft parts. A reassessment of clear cell sarcoma. *Am. J. Surg. Pathol.*, **7**, 405–413.

Dodd, S., Malone, M. and McCulloch, W. (1989) Rhabdomyosarcoma in children: a histological and immunohistochemical study of 59 cases. *J. Pathol.*, **158**, 13–18.

Doshi, R. and Fowler, T. (1983) Proximal myopathy due to discrete carcinomatous metastases in muscle. *J. Neurol. Nurosurg. Psychiatry*, **46**, 358–360.

Enzinger, F.M. and Dulcey, F. (1967) Proliferative myositis: a report of 33 cases. *Cancer*, **20**, 2213–2223.

Enzinger, F.M. and Shiraki, M. (1969) Alveolar rhabdomyosarcoma: an analysis of 110 cases. *Cancer*, **24**, 18–31.

Enzinger, F.M. and Smith, B.H. (1976) Hemangiopericytoma: an analysis of 106 cases. *Hum. Pathol.*, **7**, 61–82.

Enzinger, F.M. and Weiss, S.W. (1988) *Soft Tissue Tumours*, 2nd Edition, C.V. Mosby, St Louis.

Evans, H.L., Soule, E.H. and Winkelmann, R.K. (1979) Atypical lipoma, atypical intramuscular lipoma and well differentiated retroperitoneal liposarcoma. *Cancer*, **43**, 574–584.

Fisher, E.R. and Reidford, H. (1971) Electron microscopic evidence suggesting the myogenous derivation of the so-called alveolar soft part sarcoma. *Cancer*, **27**, 150–159.

Fisher, E.R. and Wechsler, H. (1962) Granular cell myoblastoma – a misnomer. Electron microscopic and histochemical evidence concerning its Schwann cell derivation and nature (granular cell schwannoma). *Cancer*, **15**, 936–954.

Foschini, M.P., Ceccarelli, C., Eusebi, V. *et al.* (1988) Alveolar soft part sarcoma: immunological evidence of rhabdomyoblastic differentiation. *Histopathology*, **13**, 101–108.

Garger, A.M., Soule, E.H., Hewton, W.A. Jr. *et al.* (1981) Pathology of rhabdomyosarcoma. *Natl. Cancer Inst. Monogr.*, **56**, 19–27.

Ghosh, B.D., Ghosh, L., Huvos, A.G. and Fartner, J.G. (1973) Malignant schwannoma: a clinico-pathologic study. *Cancer*, **31**, 184–190.

Golding, S.J. and Husband, J.E. (1982) Radiology of soft tissue sarcoma: discussion paper. *J.R. Soc. Med.*, **75**, 729–735.

Hashimoto, H., Kiryu, H., Enjoji, M. *et al.* (1983) Malignant neuroepithelioma (peripheral neuroepithelioma). A clinicopathological study of 15 cases. *Am. J. Surg. Pathol.*, **7**, 309–318.

Heffner, R.R., Armbrustmacher, V.W. and Earle, K.M. (1977) Focal myositis. *Cancer*, **40**, 301–306.

Hirose, T., Hasegawa, T., Abe, J. and Hizawa, K. (1989) Expression of intermediate filaments in malignant fibrous histiocytomas. *Hum. Pathol.*, **20**, 871–877.

Lanham, G.R., Weiss, S.W. and Enzinger, F.M. (1989) Malignant lymphoma. A study of 75 cases presenting in soft tissue. *Am. J. Surg. Pathol.*, **13**, 1–10.

Lawson, C.W., Fisher, C. and Gatter, K. (1987) An immunohistochemical study of differentiation in malignant fibrous histiocytoma. *Histopathology*, **11**, 375–383.

Lieberman, P.H., Foote, F.W., Stewart, F.W. and Berg, J.W. (1966) Alveolar soft part sarcoma. *JAMA*, **198**, 1047–1051.

Mackenzie, D.H. (1981) The myxoid tumors of somatic soft tissues. *Am. J. Surg. Pathol.*, **5**, 443–458.

Miettinen, M. and Virtanen, I. (1984) Synovial sarcoma – A misnomer. *Am. J. Pathol.*, **117**, 18–25.

Mukai, M., Torikata, C., Iri, H. *et al.* (1984) Alveolar soft part sarcoma. An elaboration of a three dimensional configuration of the crystalloids by digital image processing. *Am. J. Pathol.*, **116**, 398–406.

224   Tumours of striated muscle and related disorders

Nakazato, Y., Ishizeki, J., Takahashi, K. and Yamaguchi, H. (1982) Immunohistochemical localisation of S-100 protein in granular cell myoblastoma.
Cancer, **49**, 1624–1628.

Pearson, C.M. (1959) Incidence and type of pathologic alterations observed in
muscle in a routine autopsy survey. *Neurology*, **9**, 757–766.

Pritchard, D.J., Soule, E.H., Taylor, W.F. and Ivins, J.C. (1974) Fibrosarcoma: a
clinicopathologic and statistical study of 199 tumors of the soft tissue of
extremities and trunk. *Cancer*, **33**, 888–897.

Reiman, H.M. and Dahlin, D.C. (1986) Cartilage- and bone-forming tumors of
soft tissues. *Semin. Diagn. Pathol.*, **3**, 288–305.

Ross, J., Hendrickson, M.R. and Kempson, R.L. (1982) The problem of the poorly
differentiated sarcoma. *Semin. Oncol.*, **9**, 467–483.

Sarnat, H., de Mello, D.E. and Siddiqui, S.Y. (1979) Diagnostic value of
histochemistry in embryonal rhabdomyosarcoma. *Am. J. Surg. Pathol.*, **3**, 177–
183.

Slatkin, D.N. and Pearson, J. (1976) Intramyofiber metastases in skeletal muscle.
Hum. Pathol., **7**, 347–349.

Weiss, S. (1982) Malignant fibrous histiocytoma. A reaffirmation. *Am. J. Surg.
Pathol.*, **6**, 773–784.

Weiss, S.W. and Enzinger, F.M. (1978) Malignant fibrous histiocytoma, an
analysis of 200 cases. *Cancer*, **41**, 2250–2266.

Weiss, S.W., Ishak, K.G., Dail, D.H. *et al.* (1986) Epithelioid haemangioendothelioma and related lesions. *Semin. Diagn. Pathol.*, **3**, 259–73.

11 Interpretation of the muscle biopsy

Although enzyme histochemical techniques are needed to establish an accurate diagnosis in many neuromuscular disorders, some diagnoses can be established without them by using formalin-fixed, paraffin-embedded material stained with HE alone or with additional slides prepared by the PAS, PTAH or van Gieson techniques. For example, typical cases of untreated polymyositis in which inflammation is prominent pose no difficulty in diagnosis, and there is similarly no difficulty in recognizing typical examples of Duchenne muscular dystrophy or muscle tumours. However, less advanced or less typical cases are more difficult to recognize without the range of techniques available in enzyme histochemistry and electron microscopy, and in some disorders, e.g. chronic neurogenic disorders, the diagnosis can easily be missed without these methods.

11.1 Is the biopsy abnormal?

In examining a muscle biopsy it is important first of all to establish whether or not the biopsy is abnormal. Even gross examination of the fresh specimen is sometimes sufficient to reveal the presence of increased amounts of fat, or of fibrous tissue, and simple naked-eye examination of the slides will also reveal such gross changes without recourse to microscopy. However, it is not always so easy to decide whether a biopsy is abnormal. For example, biopsies taken from muscles that are only mildly affected, or are clinically unaffected, may show very slight abnormalities, for example changes in fibre size or increased central nucleation. Such abnormalities may not themselves be significant since they may occur in normal individuals, especially after excessive physical training or injury to muscle. Caution is particularly important when studies of relatives are undertaken in families with inherited muscular dystrophy.

11.2   Myopathic or neurogenic?

In abnormal muscles a broad distinction between a myopathic or neurogenic process can usually be made and this is of great importance in subsequent decisions as to the specific abnormality. It may not be possible to make a more specific diagnosis but the distinction is important to the clinician concerned with establishing the diagnosis from the whole database available from other clinical and investigative methods. In some disorders, especially polymyositis and some chronic neurogenic disorders, a mixture of features of these two broad divisions of muscle abnormalities may be present, and these may therefore pose special difficulties in diagnosis. The major histological features of myopathic and neurogenic disorders are shown in Table 11.1, in the order of their diagnostic specificity. All of these abnormalities will not be found in any individual biopsy, or even necessarily in a particular disorder. For example in an acute neurogenic disorder target fibres and scattered atrophic, pointed fibres may be prominent, but fibre-type grouping and grouped neurogenic atrophy will probably not be present since insufficient time will have elapsed to allow reinnervation by axonal sprouting and then denervation of the resulting groups of reinnervated muscle fibres. Similarly, in a metabolic myopathy fibre necrosis and regeneration may be rare, but other more specific features such as ragged-red fibres or abnormalities in muscle glycogen and fat may be prominent. Central nucleation is often found in myopathic disorders, and in these disorders it may be a feature of fibres of more or less normal size. It also occurs, however, in chronic neurogenic disorders, in which it is found mainly in hypertrophied fibres and is a feature associated with fibre splitting. Fibrosis is far more common in myopathic than in neurogenic disorders but fatty infiltration may occur in the late stages of either group of neuromuscular diseases. In polymyositis, particularly chronic polymyositis, myopathic features may coexist with inflammatory cell infiltrates and with fibre-type grouping. The latter is not usually prominent, but consists of small groups of fibres of the same histochemical type.

In practice many biopsies show only minimal abnormalities, the changes shown in Table 11.1 being more typical of more advanced disease. In *mild myopathic disorders* increased central nucleation, rounded fibres, slight architectural changes in some fibres, usually Type 1 fibres, and Type 2 fibre atrophy may be the main abnormalities. Regenerating fibres may not be prominent. In *mild neurogenic disorders* small pointed denervated fibres may be seen scattered or isolated in the biopsy with little other abnormality.

Table 11.1 The histological features of myopathic and neurogenic disorders arranged in order of their diagnostic importance and specificity

Myopathic	*Neurogenic*
Necrosis and regeneration of individual muscle fibres	Fibre-type grouping and fibre-type atrophy
Increased variability in fibre size	Small pointed atrophic fibres, often dark in NADH-tr and non-specific esterase preparations
Rounded fibres	
Fibrosis	Target or core-targetoid fibres
Architectural changes in fibres	Secondary myopathic features in chronic neurogenic disorders (see Table 4.3)
Various specific morphological abnormalities (see Table 11.2)	
Type 1 fibre atrophy	Type 1 fibre hypertrophy
Type 2 fibre atrophy	Necrotic/regenerating fibres are rare
Central nucleation	Little fibrosis
Perifascicular atrophy and inflammatory cell infiltrates in polymyositis	
Fibre-type grouping uncommon except in polymyositis	
Blood vessels abnormal in inflammatory myopathies and vasculitis	

11.3   Specific morphological changes in myopathies

The common histological features of myopathies are found developed to varying degrees in biopsies of different disorders, and the particular pattern of abnormality in the biopsy is important in diagnosis. The significance of these abnormalities is indicated in Table 11.2. Various specific morphological abnormalities occur in muscle fibres in different disorders and these are of particular importance in diagnosis, although some, for example rod bodies, are often found as a non-specific feature in muscle biopsies. Only when they are present as the major abnormality can they confidently be regarded as a pathognomonic feature. These abnormalities, many of which are uncommon, are discussed in relation to their diagnostic significance below.

Table 11.2   Significance of common morphological abnormalities in muscle biopsies

Increased central nucleation
  Common in myopathies
  Chains of central nuclei in *myotonic dystrophy*
  Plump, enlarged, vesicular central nuclei in regenerating fibres
  Central nucleation in hypertrophied fibres, especially Type 1 fibres in *chronic neurogenic disorders* and *chronic* polymyositis

Necrotic fibres
  Any active myopathy, particularly polymyositis
  Muscular dystrophies
  Toxic myopathies

Ghost fibres
  A necrotic fibre consisting of the basal lamina, with only pale remnants of sarcoplasm remaining

Basophilic regenerating fibres
  Polymyositis
  Muscular dystrophies
  Recovery after acute muscle fibre necrosis in toxic myopathies

Type 1 fibre predominance
  Metabolic myopathies
  Duchenne muscular dystrophy
  Limb-girdle muscular dystrophy

Perifascicular atrophy
  Dermatomyositis

Fibrosis
  Duchenne muscular dystrophy, even at an early stage
  Other muscular dystrophies
  Chronic polymyositis
  Some chronic neurogenic disorders

Adipose tissue in muscle
  Late stage of neurogenic or myopathic disorders
  Interfascicular fat common in Duchenne dystrophy

Hyaline fibres
  Common in Duchenne dystrophy, but occasionally a feature of limb-girdle dystrophy

Fibre-type grouping
  Reinnervation in neurogenic disorders

Small pointed NADH-tr dark fibres
  Denervated fibres: common in early stage of motor neuron disease and in polymyositis

11.4 Significance of some morphological abnormalities in muscle fibres

Increased neutral fat droplets: usually in Type 1 fibres, especially a feature of primary carnitine deficiency. May occur also in Type 1 fibres in steroid myopathy, alcoholic myopathy and in scattered single fibres in Duchenne muscular dystrophy. Fibres containing increased numbers of lipid droplets are also a feature of mitochondrial myopathies, but these fibres also contain excessive glycogen.

Ragged-red fibres: a feature of mitochondrial myopathies and of ocular muscles, in which ragged-red fibres are the major abnormality. Ragged-red fibres also occur, in small numbers, in other diseases, e.g. polymyositis and limb-girdle myopathies, but other changes are more prominent in these cases.

Increased glycogen (PAS-positive material, digestible with diastase): found in the muscle glycogenoses. In McArdle's disease the glycogen appears diffusely through the sarcoplasm. PAS-positive vacuoles are prominent in acid maltase and debranching enzyme deficiency. In the former these vacuoles are lysosomal, and show a positive reaction for acid phosphatase. The glycogen content of muscle fibres is also increased in mitochondrial myopathies, and in Type 1 fibres in steroid myopathy.

Rod bodies: when found in subsarcolemmal locations, and when very numerous, especially in children, rod bodies suggest nemaline (rod-body) myopathy. They also occur in central core disease. Rod bodies are also found in denervation, polymyositis, schizophrenia and after tenotomy, and similar abnormalities occur in degenerate myofilaments in many other neuromuscular disorders as a non-specific phenomenon. In these instances the rod bodies are not usually so strikingly located in the subsarcolemmal region as in nemaline myopathy itself.

Central cores: a cardinal feature of central core disease; also found in malignant hyperpyrexia. Cores, core-targetoid and target fibres may be difficult to differentiate, and may represent different stages of the same pathological process. *Multicores* (minicores) and *focal loss of cross-striations* may also be recognized (see Chapter 7).

Tubular aggregates: an abnormality of Type 2B fibres, reported in myotonic dystrophy, hypokalaemic and hyperkalaemic periodic paralysis, and in diabetic amyotrophy.

Vacuoles: may contain fat, or glycogen, or represent fluid-filled membrane-bound spaces in the muscle fibres. Glycogen-filled autophagic vacuoles occur in acid maltase and debrancher enzyme deficiency, and fluid-filled vacuoles, derived from the tubular system of the muscle fibres, are a feature of hypokalaemic myopathies. In periodic paralysis these vacuoles contain a faintly PAS-positive, diastase-resistant material.

Lipid-filled vacuoles occur in lipid storage myopathies, e.g. carnitine deficiency, in alcoholic myopathy and in steroid myopathy. Dark-rimmed, acid-phosphatase-negative vacuoles occur in inclusion body myositis and in oculopharyngeal muscular dystrophy. Vacuolar change also occurs in distal myopathies. Other forms of storage material have been recognized in muscle tissue, but these disorders rarely cause muscular weakness and are not usually diagnosed by muscle biopsy.

Ring fibres (ringbinden): characteristic of myotonic dystrophy, but found less commonly in many other neuromuscular disorders, especially other myopathies. Ring fibres represent fibres in which several myofibrils have become displaced, after disruption, from their normal longitudinal alignment and have taken up a spiral location around the edge of the fibre. This change in location indicates the fluidity of the sarcoplasm in muscle fibres at body temperature.

Sarcoplasmic masses: in myotonic dystrophy peripherally located zones of sarcoplasm devoid of myofibrils but containing ribosomes and tubules may be seen. In some cases most of the fibres in the biopsy may show this change.

Fibre splitting: a feature of chronic myopathic or neurogenic disorders. In the latter it is characteristically found in hypertrophied Type 1 fibres.

Muscle spindles: show a characteristic abnormality in myotonic dystrophy, in which the intrafusal muscle fibres show splitting and proliferation.

Hyaline fibres: Duchenne muscular dystrophy, particularly in the early stages. Rare in other muscular dystrophies, but a few hyaline fibres are often seen in limb-girdle dystrophy. Contain excess sarcoplasmic calcium.

Moth-eaten fibres: disruption and distortion of the intermyofibrillar network, often with a whorled appearance, best seen in NADH preparations. A non-specific change particularly prominent in inflammatory myopathy.

11.5   Relation of pathological change to clinical disability or stage of disorder

The degree of pathological change in a muscle biopsy in any disorder varies not only with the degree of disability of the patient as a whole, a factor reflecting the stage of the disease at which the biopsy is taken, but with the rate of progression or healing, and with the degree of involvement of the muscle biopsied. The latter is particularly important since a biopsy of a clinically normal muscle may show marked abnormalities in many myopathies, especially in metabolic myopathies. It is therefore difficult to suggest a prognosis from study of a single muscle biopsy in myopathic disorders. In the muscular dystrophies different muscles show different degrees of involvement at any given time. For example the legs are relatively spared in facioscapulohumeral muscular dystrophy, but more severely involved than the arms in the early stages of Duchenne muscular dystrophy. In some neurogenic disorders, however, prominent fibre-type grouping may be found in muscles of virtually normal strength and bulk, implying a relatively slow progression and effective reinnervation. This is especially typical of Type 3 or Type 4 spinal muscular atrophy, and of the neuronal form of Charcot–Marie–Tooth disease.

11.6   Are sequential biopsies useful?

Repeated muscle biopsies rarely provide useful information in assessing prognosis. The outcome is usually more accurately predictable from clinical observation. However, repeated biopsy may be useful in assessing the effect of treatment in inflammatory myopathy, and perhaps in certain metabolic myopathies. In inflammatory myopathy the development of steroid myopathy is a particular hazard of management and needle biopsy of the quadriceps muscle is useful in assessing the activity of the disease and the development of this complication.

Muscle biopsy is also sometimes used in family studies of patients with genetic myopathies, especially X-linked Duchenne dystrophy, in which dystrophin studies are useful in assessing carrier status or the presence of disease in families with muscular dystrophies. In disorders without a known genetic marker, and not associated with a raised blood CK level, e.g. nemaline myopathy or central core disease, muscle biopsy may be also useful as a method of acquiring information for genetic counselling. In inherited neurogenic conditions EMG is a more useful screening procedure than muscle biopsy.

Index

Page numbers in italics refer to figures, those in bold refer to tables.